Happy
Healthy
Kids

Much Love+Light
AOW

12

Happy
Healthy
Kids

FROM CONCEPTION TO AGE 7 WITH
Australian Bush Flower Essences

IAN WHITE

inspired
LIVING

ALLEN&UNWIN

First published in 2009

Copyright © Ian White 2009

Allen & Unwin
83 Alexander Street
Crows Nest NSW 2065
Australia
Phone: (61 2) 8425 0100
Fax: (61 2) 9906 2218
Email: info@allenandunwin.com
Web: www.allenandunwin.com

Cataloguing-in-Publication details are available
from National Library of Australia
www.librariesaustralia.nla.gov.au

ISBN 978 1 74175 663 0

Internal design by Lisa White
Set in 10/14 pt Minion Pro by Bookhouse, Sydney
Printed in Australia by McPherson's Printing Group

10 9 8 7 6 5 4 3 2 1

Contents

Acknowledgments

Firstly, I wish to thank Maggie Hamilton of Allen & Unwin for initially proposing the book and her passion for wanting as many children and their families as possible to be helped by Bush Essences. Likewise Angela Rossmanith, who shared with Maggie a similar vision for the book and for all her support, helpful suggestions and wisdom.

I am very grateful to all the many people who so kindly took the time and trouble to send me their testimonials and case histories and also to all the workshop participants who so freely shared their stories and experiences. And, to Sal McGowan and Gai Hoole from my office for so painstakingly collating all the case histories.

Most importantly a huge thank you to my wonderful wife Jane Rosenson, for giving me the permission, time and space to write the book, not to mention her tremendous and invaluable love and support throughout the project.

Foreword

I owe much to Australian Bush Flower Essences. Had I not attended one of Ian White's flower essence workshops some years ago, I doubt I would be publishing in this area today. Learning about the essences opened up a whole new world for me—of a more tangible connection with the earth, greater responsibility for my physical health, and more willingness to attend to emotional issues.

As we continue to explore the intricate connection between mind, body and spirit, it is only now we are coming to understand the powerful link between emotional imbalances and physical sickness. This link is especially important for our children's health. We now know that children who are physically and emotionally happy and healthy have a significant head start to adult life, and the use of Australian Bush Flower Essences can be an invaluable part of this process.

That Australian Bush Flower Essences are now available in more than 40 countries around the world is a truly remarkable achievement and over the last two decades hundreds of thousands of adults and children have benefited from the essences. In Belarus, Electro Essence combination was given to children who had high levels of radiation contamination following the Chernobyl disaster. In just two weeks, their radiation levels fell, on average, by 43 per cent.

As Ian continues his lifelong work with Australian Bush Flower Essences, he is discovering new healing attributes of the essences that align with our needs in the twenty-first century. It is wonderful that we now have this excellent resource to enable us to explore these possibilities for our children.

Maggie Hamilton
Publisher, Inspired Living
Allen & Unwin

Introduction

The Australian Bush Flower Essences are a totally safe, simple and extremely powerful system of healing that can help bring you to emotional, spiritual and mental harmony. Their gift of healing is based on the timeless wisdom that true healing occurs when emotional balance is restored, most physical illness being the result of emotional imbalance. Bush Essences work extremely quickly on children, as children don't have as many emotional blocks and barriers as adults do.

Flower essences are obtained by extracting the healing quality from the highest evolved part of a plant, its flowers. Ancient records show that over 3000 years ago the Egyptians collected the dew from flowers to treat emotional imbalances. The Australian Aborigines have also long used flowers to heal emotional imbalances. They would also collect the dew, or eat the whole flower, to obtain the healing vibrations from the plant. The early European settlers reported that when the local Aborigines fell ill they would treat themselves by floating waratahs in water for a number of hours then drinking the water.

The earliest written European records of flower essence usage dates back to Abbess Hildegard von Bingen in the twelfth century and Paracelsus, the famous Swiss medical professor, alchemist and herbalist, in the sixteenth century. Both prepared remedies from the dew of flowers to treat their patients' emotional problems and physical ailments. Flower essences have also been widely used in Asia, India and South America for many centuries.

During the nineteenth century attitudes towards health and healing changed, particularly in the Western world, as the body was seen more as a machine that needed fixing rather than an intricate living organism requiring love and nurture. The emotional and spiritual aspects of wellbeing were also largely cast aside. So knowledge about the healing power of flower essences faded. Even the Australian Aborigines seemed to lose some of their knowledge of the healing power of flower essences.

Then in the 1930s the English physician and homoeopath Dr Edward Bach brought flower essences back into use. His Bach flower remedies, based on English flowers, became a popular form of healing. Like other great healers such as Hippocrates, Paracelsus and Hahnemann, Bach believed that good health was the result of emotional, spiritual and mental harmony. He found that when he treated the psychological imbalances in his patients, their diseases were cured.

My family and I have been practising herbal medicine in Australia for five generations. Both my grandmother and great grandmother were among the first non-Indigenous Australians to seriously study the medicinal properties of our Australian plants. I grew up living next door to my grandmother in the bush at Terrey Hills in New South Wales. As a young boy I spent as much time as possible helping her prepare herbal extracts and tinctures as well as accompanying her on regular bushwalks where she would point out specific plants and trees and discuss with me their healing qualities. During this time I came to appreciate deeply the immense healing qualities of Australian plants.

Since the mid 1980s I have been continuing this family tradition of working with Australian plants, however, I have been focusing on developing the emotional and spiritual healing qualities of our plants.

The Australian Bush Flower Essences that I have developed carry on this very long healing tradition of flower essences. Australia has more flowering plants than anywhere else in the world, and botanists claim that the first flowering plants grew in Australia. The flora is striking in colour, mostly reds and purples, and has unique ancient forms. Australia is one of the most physically and psychically unpolluted of countries, and it has an ancient, powerful energy. The flora reflects this great energy, and the flower essences made from those plants capture that spirit and vitality.

Bush Essences have gained a worldwide reputation for their extraordinary healing powers. One of the great things about them is that anyone can use them. You don't have to be medically or naturopathically trained to recognise when your child is suffering from low self-esteem, insecurity or sadness. What's more, the essences are gentle and have no side effects, making them a perfect remedy for children and babies.

Today, Australian Bush Flower Essences are being used widely throughout the world by families and practitioners, and in hospitals as well. They have gained great respect and a wonderful reputation for being totally safe, incredibly fast acting and for producing very powerful results on not just the emotional and spiritual levels, but on the physical level too.

Bush Essences are used in cosmetic ranges; they are incorporated with aromatherapy and added to massage oils and oil burners; and they are sprayed in classrooms to enhance children's learning ability and to decrease their stress at exam time. Landscape architects utilise the plants from which Bush Essences are made in their designs so as to incorporate the healing and harmonising qualities of the essences into the environments of their clients. Bush Essences are used in hospitals in Europe and South America as a viable, effective and safe alternative to hormone replacement therapy without the increased risk of breast or cervical cancer and elevated cholesterol levels. Emergency Essence is sprayed in obstetric units to help during childbirth. Orphanages in Brazil to which we donate our essences put them in the children's food and drinks. Animal rescue groups use them on their injured animals. Flight and cabin crews take them to negate the effects of air travel. The scope of Bush Essences is quite unlimited.

One of the unique features of Bush Essences is that they can easily be combined with all other healing modalities, such as homoeopathy, allopathic medicine, acupuncture, massage, counselling or chiropractic treatments. If you or your child is on any medication, you can still safely take treatments Bush Essences alongside it.

Whether you are involved as a parent, grandparent, relative, trusted family friend or practitioner, Australian Bush Flower Essences provide a wonderful system of healing for you to help the children in your care reach their highest potential. Since Australian Bush Flower Essences became available in the mid 1980s, they've been used to bring about healing on all levels for children. They help make humans more like angels, and what better way to start life?

It is my goal for every household to have Australian Bush Flower Essences so that all family members can enjoy a better quality of life. Most importantly, I want children to be brought up with Bush Essences so that they keep their hearts open and have the courage, strength and enthusiasm to follow and pursue their goals and dreams.

I am sure Australian Bush Flower Essences will bring great benefit to you and to the children you love.

Ian White

How to use this book

This is a very practical book that I hope you will use and refer to regularly. The following is a simple guide on how to use the information it contains.

The first chapter is an overview of both Australian Bush Flower Essences and the history and philosophy of flower essences. You will find more of this information throughout the text, incorporated into the sections in chapters 2 to 10 that deal with the various stages of your child's life, from before conception through to pregnancy, birth and first years.

Chapter 11 provides an outline of a very useful numerological tool I have used for many years to gain insights into a child's character.

In chapters 12 and 13, I present guidelines on how to choose and use appropriate essences, as well as providing dosage information and details of where the essences can be obtained.

Chapter 14 contains a detailed A–Z of conditions and the essences that I have found are most effective in treating them.

At the end of the book, chapters 15 and 16 go into greater detail about each of the individual and combination essences. The colour section contains photographs of the individual flowers from which the essences are prepared.

Scattered throughout the book are a number of case histories, tips for working with particular problem areas, suggestions specifically for parents and small pieces of advice that I have found helpful over the years. You will also find a number of conditions marked with an asterisk(*). These asterisks indicate that further information on this topic, along with the essences used to treat it, can be found in Chapter 14.

Finally, the back page contains the contact details for Australian Bush Flower Essences, including information about the Australian Bush Flower Essence Society.

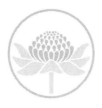

1

HOW AUSTRALIAN BUSH FLOWER ESSENCES WORK

Bush Essences help to clear any emotional and spiritual blocks you may have. Physical disease or illness is a sign of being out of balance. This imbalance first occurs on the emotional or spiritual level and if it is not addressed, it will then show up in your physical body.

For thousands of years, practitioners of Chinese medicine and Ayurvedic medicine have known that particular emotions impact specific parts of the body. For example, anger is associated with the liver, and fear with the kidney. Bush Essences promote healing and restore wellbeing by dissolving and releasing negative emotions and thoughts, and flooding your being with positive feelings such as love, joy, compassion and courage.

If you do experience an upset or a crisis in your life, Bush Essences will assist you to be aware of and listen to your inner guidance, work through your feelings and experiences, and recover more quickly.

AUSTRALIAN BUSH FLOWER ESSENCES IN ACTION

The special thing about Bush Essences is that they address and resolve the cause of a problem, rather than merely treating symptoms. An example can be seen in children in various orphanages in Brazil, to whom my company donates essences. The children used to suffer on average six or seven bouts of bronchitis each year. After twelve months of taking the remedies for grief, sadness and abandonment (the emotions which affect the lungs), that figure had dropped to less than one bout per child per year.

As the use of Bush Essences becomes more widespread, we receive more and more stories of their wonderful application and healing with children. Green Cross has found one of the combination essences, Electro, to be the most effective treatment they have used to remove nuclear radiation from the children in Belarus with the highest levels of contamination from the Chernobyl disaster. Electro reduced their levels on average by 43 per cent in two weeks, more than double their previous best treatment.

My experience with my three young boys and husband has been how nice it is to be able to get a gentle remedy out of the cupboard and treat a problem as soon as it arises. This is much better than waiting until the problem is bad enough to visit the doctor (e.g. with earaches, sore throats, conjunctivitis etc.) Then rearranging your day to visit the doctor, waiting for ages in a room full of sick people and then ending up with some harsh chemical treatment. As a family we are learning more about natural medicine and gaining greater appreciation of nature as a result. Australian Bush Flower Essences are even more special to us as we live in the bush and see many of the remedies growing around us.

Jenny Hill, New South Wales, Australia

I always ask participants in my workshops if anyone grew up being given flower essences by their parents, and though it's very uncommon to find anyone who had such a benefit, all appreciate how much easier their childhood would have been if the essences had been available to help them during all the difficult times we all experience as children. So I am particularly excited to hear of children today being brought up in families using the essences. The cases above and below illustrate how Bush Essences have been easily incorporated into daily life and become important components of wellbeing of these families.

My two-year-old son Finlay has been exposed to Australian Bush Flower Essences since the moment he was born. Boab and Fringed Violet were his first essences (apart from in utero). Now I just have to tap the bottle and he says, 'Aahh' with a big mouth open. I am just so honoured to be sharing in nature's brilliance and watch how the Bush Essences connect so well with the energies of today's special children. I am excited that one day I can pass down my experience and journey of working with Australian Bush Flower Essences to my children, so they too can experience the amazing connection with Mother Earth and the healing of themselves and others.

Sarah O'Brien, Western Australia

Throughout this book you'll find many other stories and case studies that show just how effective and powerful Bush Essences are for pregnant mothers, babies and children.

I have been fortunate enough to be aware of and able to use Australian Bush Flower Essences with my daughter since my pre-conception phase, throughout my pregnancy and birth, and during my postpartum recovery. I regularly use the essences on my young daughter Charlotte, with wonderful results. I couldn't imagine not having them as I am using them so often for such a variety of things. They are an amazing gift for us to use on ourselves and our children. People have commented to me what a truly beautiful, calm and contented baby Charlotte is, how they have never quite seen such a child. We often get told how 'lucky' we are. I truly believe that luck is not the reason she is the way she is, but a combination of our use of Bush Essences, partnered with other holistic choices we have made. The essences have made the last eighteen months of our lives with Charlotte wonderful and we look forward to continuing to use them in our family in the coming years.

Kim Mann, New South Wales, Australia

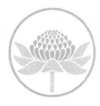

2

PREPARING FOR PREGNANCY

Making the decision to become a parent is a big step. When you and your partner are preparing for parenthood, you'll probably ask yourselves about the right time for conception. You may also have some doubts, and question whether you are both ready to take on the responsibility of being a parent or whether your relationship is strong enough to support one another through pregnancy and the years ahead.

When you do choose to try to become pregnant, it's best to allow a good two to three months to prepare yourselves before conception, as you and your baby will benefit if you are fit and strong both physically and emotionally. The effects of stress, pollution and diet can all take their toll, so a good eating and health regime is important. Bush Essences have a major role in helping you maximise your health at this time.

PREPARE YOURSELF

As you start to focus on pregnancy you might feel insecure and anxious about becoming parents. You might doubt your ability to cope, or question whether you will be competent parents. Don't worry—this is a very common response. It's helpful to build your confidence* at this time, so you feel positive and excited about raising a child.

One of the reasons you may have doubts prior to pregnancy is that you are heading into unknown territory, with many decisions to make along the way. You do, however, have the ability to make good decisions. That's why I recommend that women preparing for motherhood enhance their intuition at this time: when you take time out and slow down, you start to be more aware of what you're feeling. Your intuition is your gut feeling. When you listen to your intuition and trust it, it can be a wonderful guide and can help you in deciding on the timing of your pregnancy, for example, and in being aware of when you are most fertile. Bush Fuchsia will help you here—it is specifically for intuition, helping you to tune in and listen carefully. You'll find it in Calm and Clear Essence, Woman Essence and Cognis Essence.

Time for a second child?

We wanted to be sure about the best time to have a second child, so I took Bush Fuchsia to help me discern when our little family was ready for a new child to be born.

Maria Martinez, Argentina

TIME TO GET HEALTHY

Conception is literally about making a baby. That's why your baby's health will be enhanced when the quality of your egg and sperm is strong. You can take some very important steps to ensure you and your partner are as healthy as possible before conception.

One of the ways you can improve your wellbeing is to cleanse your body of toxins—physical and emotional. Each organ in your body is impacted by certain emotions. By cleaning out the organ concerned you also release any emotion that organ is storing. For example, your kidneys hold fear. So by cleaning out your kidneys you also release fears you may have held on to for years. And your liver holds anger, so by cleansing it you also release anger and resentment that might have built up over time. Purifying Essence is very useful here. It provides a physical and emotional detoxification for your major organs of elimination, large intestines (holding on), kidneys (fear) and liver (anger and resentment) as well as the lymphatic system. This allows you to free yourself and your baby from all the physical and emotional baggage you've been carrying.

This essence is very powerful. It clears from your body all the toxic waste from your past, regardless of how long you've been carrying it. For example, if you smoked in the past but have now given up, your body still holds some of the toxicity from the years when you smoked. I've witnessed people who haven't smoked for over fifteen years and after having Purifying Essence have had nicotine come out of the fingers they used to hold their cigarettes with. People have also had old anaesthetics, from surgery years before, released from their bodies.

Ideally I would advise you and your partner to take 7 drops of Purifying Essence when you get up in the morning, and 7 drops when you go to bed, for one month. During that time you should eat a good, wholesome diet, including lots of live food, such as fruits and vegetables, and less packaged and processed food, with no artificial colours or preservatives.

Break those habits and addictions

This can be a good time to eliminate drugs from the body. Stopping such habits as smoking or drinking too much alcohol is ideal as you want to be in the best health possible for pregnancy and parenthood.

There are three remedies in particular that will help you to give up bad habits and addictions, and they are usually combined.

- Monga Waratah gives you a sense of your own strength, and will help you accept that you don't have to stay dependent on the substance.
- Bottlebrush helps break the habit itself.
- Boronia is good for the obsessive part of addiction; for example, thinking of smoking all the time even though you may have given up. Or you may be addicted to coffee.

Take this mix of remedies for at least three weeks to help get past the habit of the addiction. I'd suggest you take the mix first thing in the morning and last thing at night, as well as any time you have a strong craving. If for three weeks you do not drink coffee or alcohol, or smoke that cigarette, this new behaviour becomes a habit. It's useful to know that anything you do for 21 days becomes a new habit, so *not* doing it also becomes a habit.

While we might not realise it, we often use addictions to cover emotional pain*. This emotional pain could be based in childhood, where you were teased or bullied, for example, or if your family home was not a happy one. Perhaps your beloved family pet died and you were heartbroken, or a close friend moved to another school. We suffer emotional pain throughout life—when we're disappointed or betrayed, when we lose people close to us, or go through a separation or divorce. To distract ourselves from the pain, or to make us feel a bit better, we can turn to drinking or smoking, or other addictions.

Once we break that addiction or habit, the emotional pain can come flooding to the surface. This is when it's useful to turn to the essences that deal with this emotional pain. Whatever the pain that's being masked, whether it's grief or sadness, anger or fear, there are specific essences to address those emotional states.

Help with giving up smoking

At a workshop, Adrianne shared that she had been a smoker for years and wanted to break the habit before she became pregnant. She took a mix of Monga Waratah, Bottlebrush and Boronia, and was able to not only stop smoking but she was also easily able to give up coffee and sugar. Adrianne followed this with Sturt Desert Pea to help her address long-held grief and sadness, which led to a lot of crying, but she said that they were 'good tears' and she felt fantastic and was releasing very old emotional pain.

Ian

Improve your digestion

A healthy diet is important in the lead up to conception and during pregnancy, especially for you as the mother, but it isn't just about eating the right food. What's also important is absorbing the nutrients from the food, and to do this your digestive system needs to be in good shape.

The digestive process starts in the mouth, so your food needs to be chewed well to break it down. Some people only chew a little bit and then swallow what is essentially unchewed food.

You may find that you have problems digesting fatty foods, or that you suffer from feelings of nausea when you eat fatty or oily foods. If this is the case for you, it could be a sign your gall bladder or liver is not working well. The remedy Dagger Hakea, which is in Purifying Essence, will improve the function of your gall bladder and liver.

Ideally, food should be eliminated within 36 hours after it's been eaten, otherwise it begins to ferment in the large intestine, or bowel. The result is that waste is absorbed through the bowel wall into the bloodstream and then goes to the liver, the big detoxifier of the body. If your liver is not detoxifying waste, especially waste coming from the large intestine, then your blood is less pure and not able to absorb as much oxygen as it passes through your lungs. Plenty of oxygen is essential for good health and vitality, so less oxygen in the blood (and therefore throughout your body) has health implications for a mother, her pregnancy and her baby. Purifying Essence will help your liver detoxify your body.

Slow down and chew

I tend to eat fast and gulp my food, but taking Calm and Clear Essence helps me to slow down and relax so that I eat more slowly. I find I don't get stomach cramps the way I used to.

Robyn Morton, New South Wales, Australia

Appreciate your body

As a mother, your growing baby will be living within your body for some months. So the more you are in touch with your body, the more aware you will be of any changes and of your body's needs. These needs start well before pregnancy, as you nourish yourself with healthy food, keep yourself hydrated with filtered water and fresh juices and get enough rest to feel refreshed and renewed.

To help you get in touch with your body and increase your energy levels, take up some form of exercise if you haven't already. The remedy Flannel Flower, in both Relationship Essence and Sexuality Essence, is very useful in helping you to appreciate your body, especially if you tend to be very sedentary and don't do much exercise. If you take Flannel Flower, you'll be more inclined to call friends to organise a tennis match rather than just sit back and watch it on television. This essence will also help you want to dance or walk, or generally move your body. Flannel Flower can also help you and your partner get back in touch with your passion and sexuality, which can be a big issue with our busy lifestyles.

Enjoying sex

When my husband saw what a difference taking Flannel Flower made to me, he started to take it too. We are both much more physical these days.

Jeannie, workshop participant, as told to Ian

Harmonise your body

Your reproductive system needs to be functioning very well for you to conceive. Woman Essence is excellent to take at this time because it will harmonise any imbalances in your body. One of its remedies is She Oak, which helps keep your ovaries healthy; in fact, the seed pod of the she oak tree is the same size as a woman's ovary.

Studies indicate that if you suffer from pre-menstrual syndrome (PMS), you are more likely to experience post-natal depression. It's really helpful to know about this link to inspire you to balance your reproductive cycle before conceiving.

To help your reproductive system regain balance, take Woman Essence for a month. Have a break for two weeks, then go back on to it for a month. Repeat this for two or three months. One of the remedies in this essence, Peach-flowered Tea-tree, also helps with mood swings and the fluctuations in hormone levels during your cycle, if this is an issue for you.

After the pill

The pill is still the major form of contraception in the Western world and has many implications for a woman's health. For example, your hypothalamus, the part of the brain that controls many functions of the body, can be seriously thrown out of balance if you take the pill for an extended period of six months or more. It's been found that Bush Fuchsia will reset your hypothalamus. It will also integrate the left and right sides of your brain, as well as your front and back brain hemispheres, enabling you to be more focused, less stressed and able to think quickly and clearly.

The heart–uterus connection

In Chinese medicine, the heart and uterus are intimately connected. If you feel happy, your uterus is more likely to function properly. Pink Flannel Flower, in Woman Essence, has a very strong action on your heart, bringing about a sense of gratitude and joy. When your heart is open, you feel joy and gratitude. This will then flow on to your uterus, enhancing conception and a healthy, full-term pregnancy.

Enhance your sexuality

Once you and your partner are in good health, you could begin working with Sexuality Essence. It will enhance the pleasure and enjoyment of intimacy between you. One of its remedies, Flannel Flower, will also help you enjoy touch during tender moments, and to talk about your inner feelings. This is ideal for couples who feel as if their shared tenderness is not as apparent in the relationship as it used to be.

Your baby will also benefit if you work with Sexuality Essence. It is a surprise to many people, but your child's belief system develops rapidly from conception until the age of three. By age three, 90 per cent of your child's beliefs have already been formed. The more comfortable you and your partner feel about your sexuality, the more likely you are to impart to your child healthy belief systems around sexuality.

Making love

To create a very intimate, receptive environment for you and your partner to make love with the intention of conceiving, use Sensuality spray. It encourages passion and sensual fulfilment.

Ian

IF YOU CAN'T CONCEIVE

Many couples imagine that they will conceive quite quickly, but sadly this is not always the case. While most couples become pregnant without too much delay, there are other couples who face disappointment month after month.

If conception does not occur when you hoped, then the male partner could begin working with Flannel Flower essence. This remedy is in both Sexuality Essence and Relationship Essence. It will increase the quantity, quality and motility of sperm.

For the woman I'd recommend Woman Essence. There are many, many case histories of women who have been trying to conceive for years who then conceive quickly while working with Woman Essence.

One of the remedies in Woman Essence is She Oak, which will help you to be emotionally open to conceive. There are a number of emotional factors that can influence or create infertility. For example, a young girl might pick up the idea from her own parents that motherhood is very hard and unrewarding. This attitude, from her mother in particular, can stand in the way of conception. One client of mine didn't want to conceive on a subconscious level because of a trauma in a past life—as a mother, she'd had to mercifully kill her six young children to save them from a brutal death at the hands of marauding soldiers. The agony of this event left such a deep scar on her psyche that she didn't ever again want to be a mother, or hold such a position of responsibility. She Oak can successfully address infertility that stems from such deep emotional causes.

A dehydrated uterus is another common cause of infertility. She Oak is brilliant here, because it will rehydrate your tissue and correct this problem while at the same time bringing about hormonal balance.

I've had over 75 per cent success rate in treating infertility with She Oak, as have many of my fellow practitioners. In fact, one medical doctor I know has enjoyed over a 90 per cent success rate using She Oak in her Sydney practice.

At an international flower essence conference in Brazil two women travelled 700 and 1000 kilometres respectively to personally thank me for making She Oak available. One had conceived within two months of taking She Oak and the other within three months. Both women had been trying to become pregnant, one for eight years and the other for seven years. They were both very moved and extremely grateful for the remedy.

Pregnant at last!

After having two babies using IVF over seven years, imagine my delight when I found I had become pregnant naturally with my third child. I had been taking:

- Woman Essence to balance my hormone levels;
- Creative Essence for creating a baby; and
- Confid Essence for confidence that my body could do it all by itself.

The essences never cease to amaze me; the power within them renews the power within us.

Sarah O'Brien, Western Australia

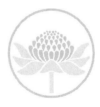

3

PREGNANCY AND YOUR BABY'S BIRTH

After trying to conceive you are now expecting a baby. Once you have an idea of when your little one will arrive, the prospect of becoming a parent starts to seem very real. This will be one of the most profound periods of your life as you nurture your unborn baby inside you for the next few months. It is a beautiful and miraculous process, and most women feel a sense of wonder and amazement at this time.

Mothers-to-be are often concerned about what they take in case it affects their unborn baby. However, one of the unique features of Australian Bush Flower Essences is that they are totally safe, so that even during pregnancy you can take them without any detrimental effect. They will help you enjoy emotional and physical balance, and this will flow on to benefit your baby.

HEARING THE NEWS

The way you react to finding out you are pregnant has a very powerful effect on your child's psyche. Even if you and your partner have been trying to conceive for a while and have been hoping month after month for good news, the actual confirmation of pregnancy can come as a shock. Even when it is joyful news, finding out you are expecting a baby can bring up feelings of fear* and anxiety*. This is a common reaction.

There are many studies revealing that children pick up on their parents' feelings from the very beginning, and these feelings can stay with them throughout their lives. When people experience age regression during hypnosis, they can be taken back to that time and remember how their parents reacted. If either the mother or father is not excited about the news, their child may experience a level of rejection and a sense of abandonment. Some parents really want their child to be a boy or a girl and may not realise that if the baby is not what they'd hoped, it will pick up on their feelings of disappointment or rejection.

If you are at all worried about your reaction to the news, then Confid Essence can be very helpful for you and your partner. It will give you confidence and help you accept the responsibility that becoming a parent brings. One of its remedies, Dog Rose, is useful for addressing any fears that come up around expecting a child, while Illawarra Flame Tree will help with any feelings of being overwhelmed by the responsibility of being a parent.

Unexpected pregnancy

If the conception has occurred before you want it, then Bottlebrush can make it easier for you, the mother, to bond with your child. For your partner, Red Helmet Orchid is the essence to help him to bond with his child. Both of these remedies are in Relationship Essence.

Ian

BE PREPARED

If this is your first pregnancy, you'll learn more and more simply through personal experience. You'll discover even more through reading about what to expect in books and on websites, asking your health practitioner questions and talking to relatives and friends who have been pregnant. You may never have been pregnant before, but you can prepare yourself as far as possible.

Take care of your wellbeing

Your wellbeing is important to you and your child during pregnancy. This includes your physical as well as your emotional wellbeing, which is affected by your relationship with your partner, the extent of support available to you and your environment. Any stress during your pregnancy will release stress hormones, which permeate the placenta barrier and impact on your baby. So it's good for you to relax as much as you can, and address any issues that might be worrying you.

Staying calm

During my pregnancy a series of upsetting things happened to members of my family. Emergency Essence helped me a lot, settling me when I was distressed.

Juanita Veaney, United Kingdom

At the same time, everyday life is full of ups and downs. Sometimes you may feel emotional, you may be frustrated by work, or you may feel tense in traffic. Rather than worrying that you're affecting your child, take steps to relax.

If there are major upsets and you feel stressed by events in your life, Emergency Essence is very helpful. It has a calming effect during a crisis. Take it as often as you need to, even as often as every ten minutes in very stressful situations.

Distress during pregnancy

Frequently at my workshops women have come to me saying how during their pregnancies a number of upsetting things had happened to them or their family and Emergency Essence had greatly helped them, settling them and easing their distress.

Ian

NAUSEA DURING EARLY PREGNANCY

A feeling of nausea can be the first sign of pregnancy. It is usually known as morning sickness*, but it can happen any time during the day. Certainly it is one of the more unpleasant aspects of pregnancy for some women.

I find that morning sickness is often associated with a mother's fear* of some aspect of the pregnancy. If you are suffering from morning sickness, then perhaps you are fearful of how your body will change shape or whether you will cope with the changes pregnancy and motherhood inevitably bring. You may fear that you won't be a good enough mother, that you won't be able to breastfeed or have enough patience or energy to look after a small baby. You might worry about your career or profession, unsure about how you will balance work and home life. You might be worried that there will be less income than before, when you were in the work force. The fears may also be vague, so that you can't pinpoint exactly what you are worried about.

Dog Rose, in Confid Essence, is the remedy for fear, and if you suffer from morning sickness you'll find that this essence will ease it. Crowea, in Emergency and Calm and Clear essences, will lessen worry.

Morning sickness

With her first pregnancy Emma suffered extreme nausea, and she was concerned it would happen again with her next pregnancy. But after starting on Confid Essence, the nausea eased and she was also feeling stronger and more confident generally.
Ian

PROTECT YOURSELF FROM NEGATIVITY

You may feel more sensitive than usual when you are pregnant. This is perfectly natural, and the good thing about it is that this sensitivity makes you more aware of anything that might hurt your baby. Being more sensitive means you are more alert; you may notice things you might not have before, and you may be more sensitive to some of the things people say.

You may find, as many women do, that when you're expecting a baby people have a lot to say to you, and much of it can be negative. A common form of this negativity is other women telling you their own or other women's horrendous birth stories. Or they may tell you tragic stories about women who experienced trauma during their pregnancy. They may think they are simply warning you or preparing you, but in fact these stories can add to any anxiety* you are already feeling.

The remedy Fringed Violet, in Emergency Essence, will give you a nice psychic protection from those people who feel inclined to share such negative stories. It is also a good remedy for general protection from people wanting to offer you all kinds of advice at this point. When you take Fringed Violet, you'll find those people wanting to tell negative stories or offer unwanted advice seem to disappear from your life altogether.

Pregnancy worries

I had a neighbour who delighted in warning me about the terrible things I'd be facing later in my pregnancy. I took Fringed Violet and now she is all smiles and very encouraging.

Vivienne Eastlake, Queensland, Australia

NURTURE YOUR RELATIONSHIP WITH YOUR PARTNER

Pregnancy is a time of enormous change for both you and your partner, and it affects each of you as individuals as well as your relationship. It is a good idea to set aside special time for each other, and to take short breaks away when you can share your feelings about the changes that are going on.

This is a momentous time for you both, especially if it is your first baby. Both of you will be thinking about how life will be different when the baby comes, and you may worry about how your relationship will stand up to the change. Bottlebrush, in Calm and Clear Essence, helps you when you are going through big changes, and I'd suggest both of you take this remedy to help you through this period.

IF MISCARRIAGE THREATENS

If there is a threat of miscarriage, or if in the past there have been a number of miscarriages, you will probably feel on edge during the pregnancy. Try to remain positive and relaxed, because this will benefit both you and your unborn baby. Keep in mind that many women have a perfectly normal pregnancy after suffering miscarriages. If there is any suspicion or sign that you may miscarry, then take Emergency Essence, which can help anything acute from happening. I've successfully used Woman Essence for a number of women who have had a history of miscarriage and was able to help them get through the first trimester when most miscarriages occur and they have gone on to have successful, healthy full-term pregnancies. Using Woman Essence throughout the first trimester can help protect you from the threat of a miscarriage.

DOUBLE OR TRIPLE THE JOY

You may feel overwhelmed if you learn that you are expecting twins or triplets. You may worry about the responsibility, about the financial and emotional burden. This is quite normal. Take the time to discuss your concerns with each other, and seek professional help if needed. Talking through worries with a professional can help you work out strategies for the future. Talk to your families and friends, too, and allow yourself to be open to any support they offer. This kind of help is invaluable, especially in those first few weeks while you are settling into a routine.

The remedy Paw Paw, in Calm and Clear Essence, will address that feeling of being overwhelmed as you contemplate life ahead raising two or more young children of the same age.

CRAZY CRAVINGS

The food cravings of pregnant women, the butt of many jokes, can be very real. You may find that you have strong cravings when you are pregnant—for ice-cream with pickles, for bread and cheese, for grapefruit.

Many cravings signal that your body needs particular nutrients at this time, and so it's helpful to listen to your own instincts. The remedy Bush Fuchsia, in Woman Essence, will help you listen to that intuition.

It could also be that your body is craving for something to which you have an allergy*. An allergen initially gives you a quick rise in blood sugar levels, followed about half an hour later by a marked lowering of blood sugar levels to a lower level than before you had the allergic food. People often don't associate the craving for the food or their drop in blood sugar levels half an hour later with an allergen. If they have that food or drink again (be it chocolate, alcohol etc.) in the short term when the blood sugar levels rise they feel better. They tend to associate feeling good—not the latter drop in blood sugar levels—with that substance. This drop leaves you feeling tired and drained. If your craving is related to an allergy, the remedies Bottlebrush and Boronia, in Calm and Clear Essence, will help to reduce the cravings. Peach-flowered Tea-tree is the essence to help stabilise problems with low blood sugar levels.

ACHES AND PAINS

Your body continues to change shape and grow with your baby during pregnancy, so there may be times when you suffer from aches and pains. Emergency Essence is a very effective remedy for pain and discomfort, especially backache and sciatica. You could ask your partner to massage Emergency Essence cream into your body wherever you feel discomfort.

Premature labour

A woman went into premature labour at 34 weeks, and the hospital kept her in bed. There was a definite urge in the mother to have this pregnancy over and done with. Subconsciously she didn't like being fat or not in control of her body. She was fearful of labour and the baby being too big in a few weeks. I prescribed her:

- Black-eyed Susan for impatience for both mother and baby;
- Dog Rose of the Wild Forces for the lack of control; and
- Bush Fuchsia to put her back in touch with her intuition, to see clearly what was best for the baby and for her.

Within two or three hours of the first dose, labour pains stopped completely and the mother was able to go home the next day. The baby was born healthy about four weeks later. It was an easy birth and the mother handled it well.

Anne Robinson, Queensland, Australia

DADS AND PREGNANCY

While you, as the expectant father, won't experience the physical changes your partner will go through directly, you will be affected by them. For example, your partner may suffer mood swings during the pregnancy, and you may not know how to respond. She may suffer nausea or extreme fatigue, and you may feel unsure about how to help her. Men often report that they feel very helpless while their partners are pregnant, and they can also feel on the outer. While your partner experiences the subtle and not-so-subtle changes day by day, you rely on information from her to let you know about these gradual changes.

A father's main role during pregnancy is to support his partner and encourage her. This is a very important role, because a pregnant woman can feel vulnerable and overwhelmed by the huge changes in her body. For example, women often feel concerned that they are gaining weight and looking unattractive, and it is helpful if the dad-to-be reassures her and lets her know that she looks attractive, and even gloriously beautiful, in her pregnant state.

A dad-to-be may generally need to increase his sensitivity towards his partner and show her greater kindness and understanding. She may be moody and snappy at times, or she may need extra affection and physical closeness. The more alert and responsive her partner is to her, the closer the relationship will grow, and the more prepared both partners will be for their baby.

For a man who wants to increase his sensitivity to and his awareness of the needs of his partner, the remedy Kangaroo Paw is excellent. Not only will it make him more sensitive, but it will help him enjoy better relationships with other people as well, though especially with his partner.

Sibling connection
Before the birth, siblings of the unborn baby can be given the essence Green Spider Orchid to help them connect with the child even before it is born. Ask them what messages they are getting from their new brother or sister, and encourage them to talk about them with you.
Ian

HANDLING BAD FEELINGS

Expecting a baby is a wonderful thing and if you have any negative feelings at all you may feel guilty about them. But every situation, however good it is, brings challenges. Pregnancy is no different. For example, you might be concerned that having the baby is hemming you in and denying you the freedom and independence you have enjoyed until now. You might worry that you will lose your identity once you are a mother, or feel frustrated your life will change and that you won't be able to do what you want to do from now on. You may direct your anger and frustration at your partner because he is not restricted or burdened in the same way as you are. These are common issues.

During pregnancy many old memories can be stirred, and so if difficult things happened when you were a child yourself they can resurface now. Just being aware of that can help you deal with any anger*, frustration*, fear* or resentment. It's best to express these feelings rather than hiding them or being ashamed of them. If you bottle them up, you're more likely to lash out at others, especially your partner.

For feelings of resentment Dagger Hakea, in both Purifying Essence and Relationship Essence, is a great remedy to help you express your feelings openly and forgive other people.

Grief

You may feel grief* during your pregnancy and not even understand why. You can feel even worse if you believe you should be constantly full of joy during these months. You are human, and pregnancy is a major life transition. Women often feel grief at these times because they are letting go of one way of life to start a new way. Often people think it's best to hold back these feelings, but it's far healthier to let them out. If you let yourself express the grief, you will emerge feeling more whole. If your partner can also go through his own process of grieving, then your relationship will move to another level of strength.

YOUR SEXUALITY

You will find labour easier if you feel comfortable with your sexuality, as pregnancy can bring up sexual insecurities or memories from any past sexual trauma such as assault, abuse or incest. Surveys suggest that as many as 70 per cent of women experience some form of sexual abuse or assault during their lives. Of course, this can affect the way you view sex and express your sexuality.

Sexuality Essence is a useful remedy for all women, whether or not they've experienced sexual abuse. Its remedy Wisteria will address any negative beliefs around sexuality. Such beliefs can develop very early, even in the womb, as a flow-on from your parents' attitudes towards sex. Wisteria will strengthen your connection to your feminine sexual energies, and will encourage spontaneous and affectionate lovemaking during pregnancy.

When your partner feels left out
A woman's partner may feel resentful because she is focused on the baby and the impending birth. If what he is feeling resembles the jealousy of sibling rivalry, the remedy Mountain Devil would help him.
Ian

BUILD YOUR CONFIDENCE

Some women lose confidence as their body changes shape. It could be that you are worried that your partner will lose his physical desire for you. You might also compare yourself with some ideal of a woman's shape that you carry. You may find that you can't think as clearly as you did before pregnancy, and worry that this state will continue.

You may lose confidence for other reasons. Sometimes worry about major life changes can have this effect. Fear* and anxiety* can erode self-confidence.

Confidence is very important for you as the birth of your child draws nearer. When you feel confident in yourself and confident that your body is doing precisely what it needs to do and that it will continue to do so, you are more likely to experience a smoother birth experience with a minimum of intervention.

Confid Essence is excellent here because one of its remedies, Five Corners, will assist you develop a sense of self-love by building confidence in your body and its processes. This combination will also help if you feel fearful or insecure, and will help you develop a positive attitude. If you feel intimidated by the medical system, for example, this essence will build the confidence to ask questions, be clear about your choices and choose the birth that feels right for you. It will also give you the confidence to follow your instincts. This is especially important as you approach labour, to know that you can behave however you want during labour without feeling guilty.

No stretch marks

A workshop participant told me how she used Face, Hand and Body Essence cream to prevent stretch marks. She rubbed it in around her belly and across her breasts during pregnancy, and found it kept her skin very elastic. The result was no stretch marks at all.
Ian

THE LAST WEEKS OF PREGNANCY

By this stage you may be frustrated or eager to have the baby now because you feel cumbersome, and you may not be sleeping comfortably. Your baby also has to deal with more physical restriction as she continues to grow in your womb. She too will feel the frustration of being in her new tiny body after her freedom in spirit form. It will be helpful to both of you if you use Wild Potato Bush, in Purifying Essence, which will give you a sense of freedom and renewed enthusiasm. You can rub the essence onto your belly so both you and your baby can benefit.

Energy boost

When I was pregnant I often felt very tired, and I found Dynamis Essence terrific. It gave me a great boost of energy.
Claire Martin, Ireland

If you're feeling impatient

It's very common for women to feel impatient towards the end of pregnancy. By this stage you may feel that you've been pregnant for a very long time and you now want to see your baby. You may also want the birth to be over and done with, perhaps because you feel anxious about labour.

There is a wonderful old expression: 'Nature is hurried at our peril'. It is a useful warning to us to allow Nature to take its proper course and to learn to be more patient and accepting.

Impatient for labour

Lynn had waited for years to become a mother and at last she was in the last weeks of her pregnancy. She came to me very edgy and irritable, unable to wait for what she called the Big Day. I gave her Black-eyed Susan for the extreme impatience. When I saw her the next week she was beaming with quiet joy. She told me she was now taking pleasure in these last weeks and was no longer in any hurry.

Anna Schwartz, Austria

When labour is near

Towards the very end of pregnancy, you may feel anxious about the labour and how you will cope. You may be anxious about whether the possibility of surgical intervention, or whether things will go as you hope or plan. You may also be worried about becoming a parent and all that entails. Whenever you feel high anxiety*, Emergency Essence will help you cope with whatever lies ahead. Take it as frequently as you need it at this time.

Being rested
During the last couple of weeks of your pregnancy, take Calm and Clear Essence to help you sleep and build up your reserves for the weeks ahead.

Ian

A wonderful touch to your baby's room is to clear it out energetically by using Space Clearing Essence, spraying all around the room a number of times before your baby comes home. You'll find your baby will sleep better and be very calm and settled in the room.

YOUR BABY'S BIRTH

Ideally, you will approach the birth of your child feeling calm and peaceful. A baby always benefits when his or her mother feels prepared for birth and looks forward to welcoming her new little son or daughter.

Pregnancy and birth are powerful experiences physically, mentally, emotionally and spiritually. These days there is plenty of information around for expectant parents and the standards of health care are generally high, but the emotional and spiritual aspects of pregnancy and birth are not well addressed. Taking into account the emotional and spiritual aspects of these mysterious, awe-inspiring and humbling experiences enables a woman to have profound growth in her life.

Time for quiet

If you have been very busy up to the labour, you may not have had much quiet time to contemplate this wonderful event. Perhaps you are still thinking of work, or are concerned about the mortgage or about what you haven't managed to finish before the baby comes. Perhaps you've only just finished work or have other children who keep you very busy.

You will be much better prepared for childbirth if in spite of all this you've taken some time to be still. You might also use this time to communicate with your unborn baby, to prepare the both of you for birth.

> **Relaxation**
> Taking Calm and Clear will help you relax, go within and be able to focus on what is happening.
> **Ian**

Prepare your environment

At the very beginning of labour, or even before it starts, it's a good idea to spray the area where you will have your baby with Space Clearing Essence. This is especially important if your baby is to be born in hospital or in a birthing centre, so you can begin labour with uplifting, nurturing vibes; you don't know what has gone on in that space before you arrived. Space Clearing Essence will purify the environment, restoring balance and creating a safe and sacred place for the new little soul to be born into. As a result, your baby will pick up on these positive energies and be more relaxed, calm and settled.

Communicating with your baby

Your baby will probably find the birth very difficult, especially as it has little control over either its tiny physical body or over the whole birth process. Many studies have shown that there is a lot of telepathic communication from the baby who is struggling to be born, and the essence Green Spider Orchid taken before and during labour will help you tune in to this and pick up what your child is trying to communicate.
Ian

Dealing with fear

It is natural for you to feel some fear* as you approach labour and childbirth. However much you are prepared, you aren't entirely sure of what's ahead. If you feel nervous, your baby will pick up on this even before he is born. Stress releases chemicals called catecholamines that travel to the placenta and on to your baby, causing him to feel your anxiety*.

It's natural to feel a bit nervous, but it really helps if you can recognise this, then slow your breathing and let yourself relax so your muscles, including the uterus and those in and around the pelvis, don't constrict and tighten, which may cause a longer, more stressful labour. The main remedy for fear is Dog Rose, which is in Confid Essence.

It brings with it courage and the ability to embrace fully this wonderful experience, and is very beneficial during labour. Emergency Essence also addresses fear and contains Crowea, which balances our muscles.

Coping in labour

As the due date for Rachel's baby was approaching, she became very fearful about labour and whether she would cope. She began taking Confid Essence the week before the due date and continued during labour. Afterwards she reported that throughout labour she had felt extremely confident in the strength of her body and mind. She was sure this had led to a smooth, trouble-free labour.
Ian

Love your body and what it does

A common attitude in our culture is that it doesn't matter what's happening inside our bodies as long as it doesn't manifest on the outside. Many women can feel this way, and when it comes to labour they can feel very uncomfortable about what their body is doing. For example, either leading up to childbirth or during labour, you may feel uneasy about the body fluids that are a normal part of labour.

An easy labour

I used the bush flowers through the pregnancy and during labour, they really helped me out. I had made three different formulas for the different stages of labour and thank God my husband was tuned in with me and the essences and was the one who suggested that I take them through labour when I didn't remember what I had put together. I had her at home and it was a beautiful birth, the labour lasted three hours and she came out very easily without having to push. I was 42 when I had her.
Juanita Gonzalez-Vasey, United Kingdom

If this is the case for you, I suggest you take Billy Goat Plum. It will help you be more open minded about the functions of your body and to accept them and feel comfortable about them. Billy Goat Plum is one of the most spectacularly beautiful of all the Australian flowers. To see the beauty of this plant is to understand how it can teach us to see the beauty in ourselves and to delight in our physical being.

Letting go

For the birth to go as easily and smoothly as possible, you have to reconnect with that primal part of yourself where you are totally uninhibited about what is going on with your body. When you are in that place, whatever your body is doing is of no concern. You are in touch with that natural, strong, feminine part of yourself as you simply allow your body to do what it knows best in giving birth. Emergency Essence will help here because one of its remedies, Dog Rose of the Wild Forces, is specifically for the fear of totally letting go. This combination provides you with the safety net of knowing you will be able to cope with whatever comes.

Getting through labour

Some labours are relatively quick, while others last much longer. There may be times during labour when you feel you may not be able to hang in there, either because you feel exhausted or that you can't manage the pain.

Stamina

Throughout my partner's labour I gave her Emergency Essence. She had previously added Macrocarpa to it to increase her stamina and endurance and to alleviate any physical exhaustion during labour.

Tom Milfenhouse, United States

Emergency Essence is invaluable throughout labour, providing effective pain relief. You can take it as often as you need to and there won't be any side effects. This essence is also very good for any birth trauma, shock or medical intervention that may occur, such as surgery or the use of forceps. It can certainly be used for any unusual complications. It is very calming for a labouring woman, and also for others around her.

Starting on the second stage of labour

Once your cervix is sufficiently dilated, your baby will start pushing down your birth canal. Gravity will help you here, so stay upright if you can. This is the second stage of labour. It can be a challenging time, and fear and pain may cause you to hold back. To help you move from the first to second stage a combination of Bauhinia, Bottlebrush and Crowea is very useful. Bauhinia helps you embrace change, Bottlebrush helps with the transition and letting go of the previous stage, and Crowea helps to relax the uterus. Keep reminding yourself that your baby will be born very soon now.

A quick pregnancy

I didn't expect it, but the first to second stage seemed to go so quickly for me. What a relief. I'd made up the combination of Bauhinia, Bottlebrush and Crowea and asked my partner to keep giving it to me.

Julia, workshop participant, as told to Ian

The crowning moment

This refers to the moment when your baby's head appears at the vaginal opening. You may be able to avoid a perineal tear if your vagina has stretched slowly enough to allow the head through. But with a first baby in particular the vagina is not very elastic, and you may need a surgical cut in the perineum to let the baby pass through. This cut is called an episiotomy, and is stitched up after the placenta has been delivered. If you need an episiotomy you will be given a local anaesthetic, unless you have had an epidural.

Emergency Essence will help here, easing any trauma caused by the stitching and anaesthetic. Take it as often as you need it. Slender Rice Flower taken after any surgery will also be important to heal the scar. Any incision, whether surgical or accidental, that's deep enough to require stitches will block the flow of any meridian through which it passes. A meridian is an energy pathway and each organ in the body has its own meridian. Slender Rice Flower is brilliant in allowing the energy to flow effectively once more along any affected meridian. It can be placed topically on the scar or taken internally and should be used for two weeks. You can even use this remedy for scars which are many years old, for almost invariably if it's deep enough to have required stitching then the energy will have been impaired along that meridian.

Forceps delivery

The birth of my first child was long and my son was delivered by forceps. I was very anxious when I fell pregnant the second time about having to go through this entire trauma again. But I took Wild Potato Bush, Dog Rose and Sundew, and when the time came for the birth it was very quick. I only used gas to help me through contractions, the expelling of the placenta, and some stitches. I was able to get up straight away and have a bath. Without the flower remedies I feel I would have had a very long and laborious labour and possibly a caesarean. I'm very grateful.

Sally-Ann Hanitzsch, United Kingdom

A caesarean delivery

These days more caesarean sections are being carried out than ever before. A c-section can be a safer procedure than a vaginal delivery in some cases but, if you are told you should have your baby this way, always ask for a clear explanation. A caesarean can be elective, which means it is planned in advance, or emergency, because the progress of labour indicates that a vaginal delivery may be unsafe for you or your baby.

If you need a caesarean section, Emergency Essence will be invaluable. It will help you stay focused despite any drugs that are administered to you, and it will ease any anxiety* or worry you have. It will also relax the muscles of your body, allowing the process to proceed more smoothly.

Healing after a caesarean

A female patient had a caesarean section eighteen months ago, however she noticed much aching in the scar on exercise, some swelling and occasional itching and redness. The swelling extended to the whole abdomen. I therefore gave her Slender Rice Flower and for 24 hours the scar felt 'strange'. Following the second dose 'a sort of tingling and aching' occurred which gradually declined as did the swelling. Two weeks on, the scar seems almost to have disappeared and the abdomen has returned to normal, the scar now being perfectly comfortable to touch. The patient is delighted.

Liz Kinsey, United Kingdom

The incision for a caesarean section cuts through about five major meridians in the body. If you have had a previous caesarean birth, then the initial scar will be reopened for this birth. It helps if you have already applied Slender Rice Flower to the scar tissue for two weeks prior to the birth to allow energy to flow along the meridians that the scar has dissected. Using it both internally and topically after the current birth will again allow the energy to flow freely along the five affected meridians.

Releasing shock or trauma

Keep using Emergency Essence after the birth, especially if there was any medical intervention with surgery, or if forceps were used. It will help to ease the shock to your system.

Ian

MEET YOUR BABY

It is a precious moment when you meet your baby face to face for the first time. It can be very emotional, seeing this little being you've waited for all this time and who is your child. For you, her parents, it is a unique moment to share together. Hold her close, look into her eyes and welcome her into the world. Your lives will never be the same again.

After childbirth

If you had pain-killers during the birth, or an epidural, or if you had anaesthetics for surgery, then you will have toxic substances in your system. Any drugs will have crossed the placental barrier, so your baby will also feel the impact of those drugs. You'll recover much more quickly from childbirth if you clear out any toxicity, and this is where Purifying Essence is excellent for both you and your baby.

For your baby after birth

You may be able to take your baby to the breast straight after the birth, but you may find your baby is not quite ready yet. She may be exhausted from the birth, or affected by any pain-killers used during labour. This will wear off, and she will soon want to latch onto your breast to feed.

Detoxing

I took Purifying Essence straight after my baby's birth to clear out the drugs I'd had, but also because it contains Bottlebrush, the essence that's specifically for mother–child bonding.

Gaia, United Kingdom

It's a good idea to dab a few drops of Boab essence onto your nipples when your newborn baby first suckles as it will help to prevent your child taking on any negative family patterns. The essence from the Boab flower is one of the most powerful healing forces I've ever dealt with, and one of the deepest acting Bush Essences. Its main healing quality is to clear the negative behavioural patterns and beliefs that are carried down from generation to generation. Negative beliefs reside in our subconscious. We are usually not aware of them but they can have a devastating influence on us for the rest of our lives, as they will influence our thoughts and conscious behaviour. Illnesses that run in families can either stem from learnt behaviour that is passed down to the children or genetically passed on. For example, if one or both parents are anxious and fearful their children are likely to have this quality. Fear affects the kidneys, so you might find that kidney stones or kidney infections are common in that family. It's not genetic, it's more learnt behaviour. Again, Boab is a specific and very effective essence for addressing both.

A midwife who worked with local Aboriginal communities in the north-west region of Western Australia—the only place where the Boab tree is found—told me that the traditional birthing practice there was for the tribe to give the pregnant woman Boab flowers if labour occurred during the flowering season. The woman would then go off by herself, dig a small hole and line it with Boab flowers, squat over it and deliver the baby into the cradle of flowers. What a wonderful gift for a newborn child—the healing, clearing the energy of Boab in his first contact with the world outside the womb.

BIRTH AND PERSONALITY

Many studies as well as extensive research by Americans Sondra Ray and Bob Mandell show that the type of birth we have has a big impact on our personality and our relationships in life. Here are some common types of birth and the possible implications for your child in each case. I also suggest remedies that would be useful for your child in addressing any negative effects arising from their birth.

A difficult birth

If your child had a difficult birth, you probably felt very stressed during labour. When a labouring mother is stressed, her body produces stress hormones which flood her baby's system. Because of the action of one of these particular hormones, a child who had a traumatic birth will continue to have a memory of what was a very disturbing experience. Emergency Essence is the one to give your child here, because it will help them process the trauma.

Breech birth

A breech birth is often difficult for the mother, and a common consequence for children born breech is that they go through life with a fear of hurting other people. The remedy Sturt Desert Rose would be beneficial in addressing this for your child, and it is one of the remedies in Confid Essence.

You often find that children born breech fear making mistakes or they can get things back to front, and this can hold them back because they aren't sure how to proceed. They will tend to ask their mothers for a lot of advice. Jacaranda, in Cognis Essence, will help all these scenarios.

Breech delivery

Kimberley was a breech baby, and as a young child she would be so afraid of making a mistake that she would choose to do nothing. She was given the remedy Kapok Bush, to help her be more willing to give things a go.
Ian

An unplanned baby

If your pregnancy was unplanned, you may find your child can be disorganised in life and have trouble planning. Sometimes these children can be a little clumsy; they can be accident prone, just as they themselves were an accident. Cognis Essence will be useful for helping to ground your child, improve his attention to detail and his coordination.

Unwanted baby

Sometimes these children feel they are not good enough and self-esteem can be a big issue—Confid Essence helps this. It's not uncommon for these people to experience a lot of rejection in relationships and in situations in their lives. Illawarra Flame Tree will help them deal with rejection. Alternatively, they may do the opposite and not let people get close to them; they are afraid of getting hurt so they will push people away. Pink Mulla Mulla addresses this aspect.

A long labour

When the labour has been very long, children can suffer from subconscious worry and guilt that they will hurt people. Confid Essence is a good one for such children because of its remedy, Sturt Desert Rose, which will address feelings of guilt. Like breech babies, they can feel that life is tough and a struggle, and sometimes this carries over into their relationships. Sunshine Wattle can also help here, giving a sense of optimism about the future and acceptance of the beauty and joy in the present moment. Sometimes they can be late bloomers, and have either a little physical or emotional immaturity. Kangaroo Paw will help with this.

Forceps birth

With forceps births, sometimes children can develop the belief that they can't make it on their own. They can feel dependent on others. Monga Waratah will help them break this dependency and find their own power. Kapok Bush helps them not to give up just because they find things too hard or think they can't do it.

Sometimes these children feel that their head and their heart are disconnected and separate, and Hibbertia is a wonderful remedy for this feeling. In fact, this is a shrub with yellow flowers, and when the petals fall from the stem little yellow hearts are left lying on the ground under the bush. Yellow represents the intellect in colour therapy, and the plant's visual message, what is known as the Doctrine of Signatures, indicates the reconnection between the head and the heart.

Caesarean birth

With a caesarean, not only is there the surgical intervention, but also the anaesthetic that passes through to the baby. There is some similarity to forceps delivery in that these children are not directly involved in the process; external forces are acting upon them. A caesarean-delivered child may always want to be in control. Hibbertia will help settle such children. Or they might be the ones who like to jump in and take charge of situations—if you find this to be a problem, use Gymea Lily.

Because they have not gone through the birth canal, caesarean-born children can often have a strong craving for physical touching and for a lot of affection. Flannel Flower, in Relationship Essence, will help address this.

These children may find it difficult to make decisions because the birth decision was made by someone else. The remedy Paw Paw, found in Cognis Essence, will help a child who feels overwhelmed and can't make up his mind.

Caesarean babies

Children born by caesarean section can have a hard time completing things because they didn't have a 'complete' birth (i.e. it was done for them) so the remedy Jacaranda, in Cognis Essence, will help them to finish what they start.
Ian

Cord around the neck

Babies born with the umbilical cord around their neck are obviously going to need Emergency Essence, which contains Fringed Violet for shock and trauma. Being born like this can be life-threatening and very frightening for everyone involved.

These children can be hypervigilant, feeling that the world is not safe. They are always on guard and can't relax. Hibbertia is the remedy for this.

As they grow older, these children can recreate both dramas in their relationships and even life-threatening events. There can be a sense that they enjoy the drama and like being the centre of attention. In this case, Gymea Lily is the remedy.

Alternatively, such children can feel smothered in relationships, as if they are being strangled. The remedy Flannel Flower, in Cognis Essence, is good for establishing healthy boundaries and the feeling that it is safe to be with others.

A baby of the 'wrong' gender

These days many parents find out the gender of their child well before the birth, but some choose to wait until the birth to find out. Some are disappointed or 'thrown' by the gender of their baby whenever they find out. Even if parents quickly recover from their disappointment, a child will energetically pick up on their parents' first reaction.

One of the most common consequences of this experience is the child's sense that he is not good enough. These children can have low self-esteem and feel they are not acceptable as they are. Confid Essence will help here, especially since it contains Five Corners, an essence I regard as possibly the most important for children. It specifically addresses low self-esteem and lack of confidence.

Puberty can be a very difficult time for these children as their bodies sexually develop and their gender becomes very apparent. This can bring up earlier, old wounding emotions such as guilt because they weren't what the parents wanted, or shame about their body; secondary sexual characteristics such as growth of breasts, facial or pubic hair can bring up strong feelings of guilt and shame for them at puberty. Adol Essence addresses these emotions and helps your child go through these major biological changes.

Self-assurance

My partner was sure we were having a boy, so when our daughter was born he was shocked, although he loved her right away. I was aware of how she might be affected by any disappointment he had, so I gave her Confid Essence when she was little. She's now a really easy-going, self-assured little girl.

(Name supplied but withheld on request)

Twins

The first-born of twins often assumes more of a leadership role, and if this is overly pronounced then Gymea Lily can help them step back and not always have to be the boss. The second twin tends to be more of a follower, and the remedy Dog Rose will allow them to step forward more, to be seen for who they are rather than just tagging along.

If there is a lot of sibling rivalry, or if the twins are very competitive by nature, then Mountain Devil will help with this, allowing them to accept each other. Twins are often very conscious of their own space, and a have a need for it. Consequently, Flannel Flower will help them to develop sound boundaries in relation to this.

Down syndrome

Down syndrome children (and other children such as those born with an umbilical cord around their neck which has blocked off circulation to the brain and resulted in permanent brain damage) are usually having their first incarnation. They've come here to Earth to be observers. What they require is a lot more security, love and safety and a very strong connection to their parents.

Bonding is going to be very important for these children. The remedies Bottlebrush and Red Helmet Orchid will help them establish strong bonds with their mother and father. Parents can also take these remedies to help them bond with their child. These children can be more susceptible to trauma around them so Fringed Violet, which can be taken regularly, offers a nice protective energy.

A calm environment
A sense of peace and calm is important for children with Down syndrome, so Calm and Clear Essence can be a useful remedy as they are growing and developing.
Ian

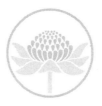

4

THE FIRST FEW DAYS

At last, after all these months, your baby is safely delivered. You've been through a powerful experience physically, emotionally, mentally and spiritually, and you may find you feel a bewildering mix of emotions. There's the elation of having given birth to this new little being and the wonder of it all. You may also feel exhausted and flat after the huge effort of giving birth. However you feel, share it with your partner and know that yours is a normal response. Be gentle and patient with yourself.

HANDLING YOUR BABY

Many new parents feel nervous about handling their newborn, especially if this is their first baby. You may fear that you'll be clumsy with this fragile little being, although in fact tiny babies are quite robust. You may be worried that you don't know how to hold your baby, or that you won't know how to attend to her needs. The remedy Bush Fuchsia, in Calm and Clear Essence, will help your coordination, and it also works on intuition. You'll feel more in tune with your baby and more confident that you know what she needs. Of course, it's a good idea for dads to take it as well, because they can feel nervous about holding and handling a small baby too.

Creating a harmonious space

During our five-day hospital stay after my daughter was born, I would regularly spray Space Clearing Essence around the room before and after visitors to keep the energy kind to our new little one. As a result you could feel the stillness and harmony in the room. It felt safe and warm, and people would often comment on what a nice room it was. In fact it was no different to any other hospital room except for its lovely calm energy.

Kim Mann, New South Wales, Australia

A 'FLOPPY' BABY

All babies are a little 'floppy' at birth, but if your baby is particularly floppy or slow and sluggish, it could be due to drugs you took during labour. It could also be due to smoking tobacco or other drugs during pregnancy. Emergency Essence is the remedy to initially use here. It contains the remedy Sundew, which will bring your baby quickly into his body, grounding him and allowing him to be fully present. Together with Sundew, your continuing love for your baby will bring his soul into his little body. If your baby was exposed to drugs, then consider giving him Purifying Essence for two to four weeks once Emergency Essence has initially settled him.

BONDING

That early bonding between a mother and her baby is very important, and breastfeeding provides the best way of bonding. When you breastfeed the hormone oxytocin, which is known as the 'love drug', floods your body so that you feel a strong, loving connection with your baby. Some new mothers don't feel an overwhelming love for their baby just after birth, and they worry they are not feeling the way they should be feeling. The intensity of labour can leave a mother feeling deflated, and breastfeeding will help her to nurture a natural love for her tiny baby.

It's been found that if a baby is not put to the breast within the first six hours after birth, it will affect the bonding between mother and child. A common reason for a baby not going to the breast very soon after birth is trauma during birth. It could also be that the baby is premature and needs to be put into a humidicrib.

Over the years many women have told me in my workshops that they have noticed the difference when they've had a child who did go to the breast within those first six hours and another who didn't. They report that there is always far healthier bonding when the baby is breastfed soon after birth. Many have told me that they gave birth twenty or 30 years ago and they still don't feel they have as strong a bond with the child whose breastfeeding was delayed after birth. The wonderful news for these women is that even years after the birth you can take the remedy Bottlebrush to improve the mother–child bond. I'd recommend that both mother and child take the remedy.

Overcoming a child's anger

A mother brought her three-year-old daughter to me for help. The mother told me that she and her daughter had never connected and the little girl seemed to have a lot of anger towards her. I picked up that the girl had been unhappy in the womb. I asked her if she liked being a baby and with a look of delight in her eyes she replied 'yes'. I then asked if she liked being inside Mummy's tummy, and her whole energy changed dramatically. She yelled: 'No, I kicked and kicked, I hated it and I wanted to get out.' Her face was red and her anger level had shot up.

Her mother, sitting in on this session, was stunned. She told me she had not wanted the child and was very angry at being pregnant. In the womb, the baby had felt and accepted this energy and taken it on as her own. This had created an energy block in her body, and she had been operating from this energy block since that time.

The little girl then chose her own Australian Bush Flower Essence cards and I prescribed the essences she chose: Bluebell, Grey Spider Flower, Red Lily, Silver Princess and Bottlebrush. Three weeks later the girl's mother was elated as she reported that they no longer argued over everything. Her daughter was a much happier child in general.

Maggie Landman, Queensland, Australia

It is much easier for a woman to bond to her child than it is for a man. The baby develops within her, they shared the same hormones and blood supply, there is also the 'love' hormone oxytocin and breastfeeding to help that bond. However, poor bonding between mother and child may occur if the mother didn't want to have the child, for whatever reason. Again, Bottlebrush can be used to forge that bond and Dagger Hakea for any resentment the mother may harbour, while for the child consider Tall Yellow Top for any sense of abandonment or alienation. Red Helmet Orchid assists the bond between fathers and their children and will be discussed at length later in the book.

BREASTFEEDING YOUR BABY

Breast milk is the best food for your baby because it contains the perfect balance of nutrients he needs during the first few months of life. What's more, breast milk is always the perfect temperature and it is always readily available. It is easy for your baby to digest and it protects him against infection and possibly even allergies. You'll find that a baby who is breastfed has softer stools and they don't smell badly, an indication of how well the milk is digested.

Immediately after birth your breasts produce colostrum, a clear fluid with a concentration of nutrients and antibodies for those first few days. Your breast milk will come in around the third or fourth day after birth.

Developing physical intimacy

A child may have more difficulty with physical intimacy as a result of not going directly onto the breast following birth and having that initial warm, nurturing contact with his mother. The remedy Flannel Flower, in Relationship Essence, will help a child develop ease with physical intimacy.

Ian

Make sure you are sitting or lying comfortably when you breastfeed, and that your baby has correctly latched onto your nipple. New mothers often wonder how long their baby should feed. A general rule is ten minutes on each breast, but some babies suckle for less time than this. If your baby falls asleep at the breast after taking milk only from one side, at the next feed start him on the other breast. It is unlikely your baby will be underfed; as long as he continues to put on the correct amount of weight, he is doing well on breast milk alone.

Peaceful breastfeeding

Charlotte was given Boab, Bottlebrush, Sundew and Fringed Violet before her first breastfeed and then for the first six weeks of her life. I would rub it onto her fontanelle, wrists and temples daily when I felt it appropriate. I found that she seemed very content and at peace each time I'd apply it and she'd often settle into a very peaceful state, be it asleep or awake. I have since used Angelsword and Fringed Violet for any time I felt she needed some protection.

Kim Mann, New South Wales, Australia

The more relaxed you are about breastfeeding, the easier you will find the whole process. And the more you breastfeed, the more milk you will have. If you 'top up' the breast milk with bottled milk, you'll find that your baby may suck less strongly at the breast and the amount of milk you produce will diminish.

Focused on feeding

From birth to the third year nutrition is essential for the child. What is fed to the child is important, as is how it is fed, under what circumstances it is fed and if there is love when it is fed. Many women have mentioned that by using Calm and Clear spray or drops they have been able to let go of other distractions around them, and be very focused, still and loving while feeding their baby. Women talk of both they and their child being very centred and very still together.

Ian

You may find that as you breastfeed you experience mild contractions of the uterus. Breastfeeding encourages these contractions, allowing your uterus to return to its pre-pregnancy shape. One of the other benefits of breastfeeding is that it helps you burn off any fat you may have put on during pregnancy.

Enjoying breastfeeding
Women who were not breastfed themselves can experience some repugnance at the idea of a baby suckling at their breast. The essence Billy Goat Plum will help a woman who doesn't like the idea of breastfeeding; it allows her to accept her body and come to enjoy its wonderful functions.
Ian

Treating mastitis

While I was breastfeeding, the glands in my breasts became inflamed, causing mastitis. I took Woman Essence each day to harmonise any imbalances, and I added Bush Iris which works on the lymphatics. There are lots of lymphatics in the breasts. Also, I rubbed Emergency Cream into the breast area. The mastitis settled quickly.

Eva, address withheld on request

PROTECT YOUR BABY

In some cultures, newborn babies are not taken outside the home for six weeks after birth, and the parents are very careful about who has contact with them. A baby's aura is open during the first six weeks, and keeping them indoors allows for the development of the baby's psychic protection and emotional wellbeing.

However, you can close off your baby's aura by gently rubbing a few drops of Fringed Violet over his soft spot, known as the anterior fontanelle, and making the sign of the cross. To locate this soft spot, rest the base of your baby's palm gently across the bridge of his nose and note where his middle finger ends. Once your baby is protected in this way, you don't need to worry so much about who comes into contact with him or when you can take him out. This is especially useful if your baby is born in a hospital, where there are many different people who either work or visit there.

WHEN YOUR NEWBORN CRIES

You may find that your baby cries often during her first week for no apparent reason. You've fed her, you've changed her and you've cuddled her, but still she cries.

Notice whether she cries each day around the same time she was born, because this is when she is reliving and processing the birth experience. This is especially the case if the birth was difficult because, if you are stressed during labour, stress hormones flood both your system and the baby's. The hormone oxytocin helps the uterus contract, and it also has an amnesiac effect on your baby so that she has no memory of the birth. But this effect can be blocked by the stress hormone ACTH and newborns who have had traumatic births have a full memory of it. Fringed Violet will enable a baby to process and release trauma from the birth experience.

Settled baby

A young mum and her baby had a difficult, long birth, which eventually meant an epidural. The baby is now three days old and very unsettled. However, when drops of Fringed Violet are placed on the baby's crown, the baby settles down quickly and goes to sleep. The mum is very happy with the results.

Salliane McGowan, New South Wales, Australia

FEELING DOWN

During those first few days, you will be recovering from the birth and starting to breastfeed your new baby. You may find that, three or four days after the birth, you become weepy and emotional. This is often called the 'baby blues' and is caused by hormonal changes. Usually the baby blues last just a few days, and during this time you need reassurance and support from your partner. Remember that you have been through a powerful experience, and you now have responsibility for a tiny new being. This realisation can be overwhelming, and can contribute to the weepiness.

Some women find that they continue to feel down, and these feelings may even get worse. In this case, she may be suffering from postnatal depression. There are a number of reasons for a woman to suffer some postnatal depression. For example, she is more likely to experience it if she doesn't have good family support. If a woman experienced a poor relationship with her own mother, if there was a lot of trauma in childhood or perhaps physical or sexual abuse, then statistics indicate she is more likely to suffer from postnatal depression than a woman who had an easier childhood. A woman with a difficult beginning is more likely to lack the confidence to be a good mother.

You may feel down because you are finding it difficult to let go of your old roles. For example, perhaps you've had a successful business career and now you want to focus on being a mother. Or perhaps you are worried about how you will juggle your new role as mother with your professional career. You may have other children and are worried about how you will cope once you go home.

Helping to cope

I used Emergency Essence three times a day for a week after Finlay was born and never had the day-3 emotional meltdown.

Sarah O'Brien, Western Australia

Postnatal depression

If you continue to feel very down after childbirth, you'll find that Waratah, in Emergency Essence, is a very powerful remedy for bringing you back into balance at this time, while Tall Yellow Top is specific for loneliness, alienation and depression also.

Ian

Woman Essence is excellent for a new mother. It includes the remedies Bush Fuchsia, Pink Flannel Flower and She Oak, which will help settle your hormones after the birth, and Bottlebrush, which will help you let go of your old roles, giving you the ability to cope with change and attend to your new role as mother while aiding your bonding with your new child.

HEALING SCARS

If you had a caesarean section, an episiotomy or tearing, take the remedy Slender Rice Flower or rub a few drops of it onto the scar to help it heal very quickly and ease any tenderness. It will also clear any blocking of your body's meridians caused by the tear or incision. Two very powerful meridians that work on the nervous system begin in the area around the perineum, so proper healing is important.

Scar tissue can be stronger than steel, and I've seen people develop adhesions after surgery which are then often removed by further surgery, but the problem just keeps repeating. Women who have had caesareans can develop these adhesions, and Slender Rice Flower will help dissolve them.

ADVICE FROM OTHERS

New mothers often feel they are the target of advice from other people about what they should be doing for their child. Sometimes it can seem that everyone thinks they are an expert on newborns and childrearing! Many people have ideas about how babies should be handled and how children should be raised, and they aren't afraid to voice their opinions.

If you feel overwhelmed by all the suggestions and warnings that people like to offer you, Fringed Violet, in Emergency Essence, will be very useful. It offers psychic protection from all the advice, suggestions, even negativity that other women—often strangers—can be so keen to pass on. So many women have reported that these women just 'disappear into the woodwork' after taking Fringed Violet.

Too much advice

I was feeling unsettled by all the advice my mother-in-law was passing on to me, and other older women in the family too. I took Fringed Violet to protect myself, and I followed it up with Bush Fuchsia, in Woman Essence. It helped me to trust and follow my own natural mothering instincts. I felt such a relief.

Lesley Johnston, New South Wales, Australia

THE SOUL CALL

It can help parents to know that a soul chooses their particular incarnation and knows what is going to happen for the first twelve years of life. This means that before a child is born, its soul knows what's ahead: they know, for example, that their mum is going to have a serious health problem in a few years; or that mum and dad are going to split up when the child is four years old. They know all these things, and they've chosen them for this life.

If a soul flags a particular situation and plans to be born into it, it may change its mind at the last minute. In this case you'll have a second soul who has been watching and they'll take the position instead. It may not be the most ideal set-up for this soul, but it's a real privilege to have a physical body and to be on the Earth plane. You could say there's a queue for this, so the soul says, 'It isn't ideal for what I have to learn and experience, but I'll take it anyway.' Usually this is the case if there are a lot of problems around the birth and during the first eight weeks of the baby's life. It is not a smooth transition.

If a child is stillborn or passes away in the first eight weeks of life, it usually means the conditions haven't been right for that soul coming in. If a child lives past the first eight weeks and dies before the age of thirteen, it is usually their last incarnation. They have come to Earth to be of service. We think of this as a great tragedy, and on the human level it is, but for the life of that soul it's a very valuable experience.

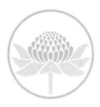

5

THE FIRST YEAR

The world is new and strange to little ones who have just arrived. They spend their first weeks and months getting used to their surroundings and learning how to interact with their environment.

During the first year of your baby's life your little one will grow from a tiny, vulnerable newborn child to an inquisitive one year old. You'll be amazed at how your baby grows and develops, and you'll also be amazed at how busy you are as you look after this little person and attend to her needs. Parents who expect life to go on the same as before baby came are usually in for a big surprise. Adults may follow timetables and be fairly predictable, but babies have different ideas.

MAKING ADJUSTMENTS

Your baby will also have to make adjustments to this new life. Pink Flannel Flower is a beautiful essence to give to babies to help them adjust. The flower itself has an intense pink centre and is all about heart energy, and the essence has a great affinity with babies whether they are in the womb or in their first five years of life. Pink Flannel Flower keeps their heart chakra open with the high love vibration they came to Earth with, and helps them to adjust to the realities of life on Earth.

The powerful love energy they have is very healing to people around them, helping others to open their hearts and be unafraid of love.

Relaxed, calm baby

My baby is very calm and relaxed, and nothing seems to faze her. I put it down to taking Calm and Clear Essence and a variety of Bush Essences throughout my pregnancy. I use the spray in our home and regularly in Charlotte's room. I have found this creates a lovely energy which can really help build a calm and quiet space, especially while breastfeeding and in general quiet, wind-down time. Charlotte seems to stop/slow down in its mist and you can see her whole body relax, calm in the centre.

Kim Mann, New South Wales, Australia

TOUCH AND MASSAGE

Touch is a basic need of all human beings. In fact, it's important for survival. Many years ago researchers found that baby monkeys who were deprived of touch died soon after birth, and human beings are no different. We need to be cuddled, held and stroked from the very start in order to thrive.

When you touch your baby you are also bonding more deeply with her. Don't believe the theory that you can spoil a baby by cuddling her too much. In that first year of life babies learn a lot about loving relationships from their parents in the way they offer plenty of physical affection.

Babies love to be massaged, and it's a wonderful way to calm a baby who is a bit unsettled or cranky. It is also a wonderful way to feel more relaxed yourself. After your baby's bath is a nice time for a massage, and you could add a few drops of a favourite Bush Essence to some baby oil to bring a calming, gentle energy to you both. Using your fingertips, slowly and gently stroke her little body, from her face, neck and shoulders down to her ankles, feet and toes. Gaze at her as you massage her, and sing quietly or talk to her in a low voice as you go. You can certainly use any of the five Bush Essence creams or even make your own cream by mixing 7 drops of a Bush Essence stock to 1 tablespoon of cream or oil.

SOOTHING YOUR BABY

Your baby depends on you for his survival, and how much attention and care you give him will have an impact on him for all of his life. He will learn early the basics of good relationships, and that includes a loving response when he needs you. Always respond to him when he cries, and don't worry that you are spoiling him if you cuddle him when he is unsettled. When he is a tiny baby crying is the only way he can communicate, and answering him is a way of showing him he is important to you and that his needs matter.

It can be very trying for parents when a baby cries persistently. Your baby may become fretful in the late afternoon and evening, and nothing you do seems to soothe him. Do what you can to remain calm, because babies do pick up on your tiredness or impatience. Calm and Clear Essence in mist form sprayed around the room will help you remain patient and unruffled, and will also settle your baby.

To soothe your baby, you could try holding him up against your shoulder and gently rubbing his back; or rock him gently either in your arms or in his pram; or try lying him across your lap and stroking his back and legs.

DAD'S ROLE

A father's main role at this time is to support his partner. During the first three years of your child's life her main relationship is with her mother, and if you, as father, can do what you can to support your partner, then your baby and her mother will be able to bond more effectively. As a result, your child will be more secure and more confident.

While your baby will be the focus of your partner's attention for some time, it is important that you and your partner make some time for each other. Some men feel very left out and miss the love and attention they enjoyed before the baby arrived. Encourage your partner to share with you her observations of your baby.

The main time for deeper bonding between a father and his child is when the child is between four and seven years of age. However, for the first time in any culture, we are now seeing men being present at the birth of their children. French birthing pioneer

Dr Michel Odent, who along with Frederick Leboyer revolutionised birth techniques, was unable to find any record of men being present at the birth of their children, in any culture, in any previous period of time. Of course, a man doesn't have the same biological experience as his partner does. He doesn't have his child develop within him energetically and physically, and he doesn't have the experience of oxytocin flooding his body as the mother does. However, being present at the birth does seem to help a man develop a particular bond with his baby.

Father and child bonding

If as a father you feel disconnected from your baby, the remedy Red Helmet Orchid will help you bond with her. It will help you recognise that you need to spend time with your family and establish a strong, healthy bond.
Ian

COLIC

If your baby cries after feeding, pulling his legs up in pain, he may be suffering from colic*. You'll find the remedies Crowea and Paw Paw very useful in this case. Both remedies are found in Calm and Clear Essence, and will work on the stomach to help your baby's digestion.

Dealing with colic

For acute colic pain, rub a little Emergency Essence cream around your baby's abdomen.
Ian

Your baby may suffer from colic if you are feeling tense as you handle him and breastfeed him. You could take Calm and Clear Essence yourself to keep you calm and relaxed while you are breastfeeding and attending to your baby.

Relieving colic

James was born six weeks prematurely. Five weeks after birth he started pulling his legs up and screaming after his feed for an hour or more. His mum had switched to formula milk soon after he came home from hospital. I saw him at ten weeks old, and thought the colic could have been due to an immature digestive system and the change to cow's milk formula. I prescribed a bottle of Emergency Essence to which I added Paw Paw. I told his mum to rub it on his tummy and to rub 1 or 2 drops onto his gums morning and evening for a week. Should he have a colic attack, she could repeat this process every ten minutes until the symptoms subsided. After a week he was much more settled and alert, having only a few short attacks. Two weeks later his colic had stopped, he'd put on weight and his complexion had changed from being dark and red to more peaches and cream. His nightmares also stopped. It was great to see such a dramatic change! ABF essences are amazing!

Sally Middleton, New South Wales, Australia

YOUR BABY'S SLEEP

Some young children sleep well and some don't. Parents often feel anxious if their child is not a good sleeper, believing it's because they are doing something wrong. They hear other parents talking about babies who sleep through the night and judge themselves harshly. But this is not useful, because it will only make you more anxious and your baby will pick up on this.

If your baby isn't sleeping well, she may need closer contact with you. Sleeping in the same bed can be a very good thing for your baby. You may worry that you will roll over and crush your baby, but this is an incredibly rare possibility because parents have a natural intuition and you are more sensitive to your baby's presence than you may realise.

Sometimes your child will pick up on energies in the room. She may sense spirits, for example, and feel unsettled. This is where spraying Space Clearing Essence is useful.

It will clear the room out energetically. Spraying this essence can be enough to allow your child to feel more comfortable and thus go off to sleep.

For parents: Desperate for sleep

It is common for new parents to be deprived of sleep and to stumble through the day feeling exhausted. Dynamis Essence will give you energy in the morning and renew your enthusiasm for each new day.

You may be so tired that even when your baby is sleeping you are unable to fall asleep and get good quality sleep. In this case, Calm and Clear Essence will help you make the most of the opportunity to sleep. It is available as a spray, as drops, or as a cream for your face and hands. Because it contains Black-eyed Susan, it will also help you if you feel impatient because your baby won't go to sleep.

Ian

THE PAIN OF SEPARATION

Babies start to suffer separation anxiety* around the age of six months. You'll find that your baby may become distressed if you walk away or leave him with someone else, even if he knows that person. Your baby will feel more secure if you always respond to him when he cries or calls for you, and if you let him see that when you leave the room you always return to him. This way he'll trust that you will not abandon him.

The adopted child

The earlier any trauma associated with feelings of abandonment and rejection are dealt with, the less likely adopted children are to act out at puberty. Statistics show that adopted children go through a more turbulent time at puberty than children who are not adopted. Tall Yellow Top is a good remedy for the adopted child. It specifically addresses any sense of abandonment, and will give a sense of belonging. Use Bottlebrush and Red Helmet Orchid for bonding too.

Ian

PRIMITIVE REFLEXES

During your pregnancy and in the early months of life, your child is protected and assisted by reflexes. These are controlled by the brain stem, the oldest part of the central nervous system, which is found just above the spinal cord. The reflexes are involuntary responses to stimuli such as touch, noise, heat or internal stimuli such as thirst and hunger.

During the time in the womb the higher centres of the central nervous system are not yet fully developed, so your baby needs what are known as 'primitive reflexes' for survival and also for development. However, by the time your child is twelve months old, the higher centres of her central nervous system are mature enough for her to have more conscious control of these activities, and the primitive reflexes start to fade.

The primitive reflexes develop and fade in a very specific order, and are integrated in specific sequences. If this doesn't happen, it can cause extra stress on the central nervous system. This can affect your child's coordination, concentration, temperament and learning ability.

There are about twelve major primitive reflexes, one being the palm reflex. If you stroke your baby's palm, she will automatically clasp your finger. If she retains this reflex beyond the first few months of her life she may have difficulty with fine motor coordination later on, such as holding pencils or scissors.

The main reason that primitive reflexes either go out of sequence or are retained is some form of trauma during the pregnancy or the first few months of life. It might be physical trauma, such as a car accident or a bad fall; it could be due to exposure to toxic fumes, such as cigarette smoke; it could be emotional trauma, such as the death of someone close to the mother. However, one of the major traumas is birth trauma. For example, for a child born by caesarean section the experience is like being woken by a tremendous clapping of cymbals over your head.

Any problems with primitive reflexes can be addressed effectively with Bush Fuchsia. There may be a genetic predisposition to the retaining of primitive reflexes so, if trauma does occur, some children are genetically more susceptible to its effects. Where this is the case, the remedy Boab can be used to address this family pattern. Obviously, if there has been severe trauma Emergency Essence would be used first to help release the trauma and to stop it from being stored in the body on a cellular level.

A 'floppy' baby

My grandson Benjamin was born with the placenta wrapped around his neck; he was a 'floppy' baby, and wasn't developing at a normal rate and had no coordination between the top and bottom of his body. He also had a lot of muscle weakness and was ten months old when I treated him. I prescribed Emergency Essence as well as:

- Sundew for grounding;
- Tall Yellow Top for a sense of belonging;
- Crowea for muscle strength; and
- Bush Fuchsia for coordination.

After four days there were improvements, he was reaching for things; after seven days he sat up on his own when propped up, and after three weeks he was laughing and beginning to develop normally. He is now five years old and a happy, healthy child.

Patricia Ralph, New South Wales, Australia

CURING CRADLE CAP

Cradle cap is a skin condition that can affect a baby's scalp, causing crusting and scaling. It usually appears during the first three months of your baby's life. It is very common and your baby won't be bothered by it, but it may bother you.

Cradle cap can be treated with Green Essence. Mix 7 drops of stock with 30ml of water and gently spray it onto the affected area morning and night for up to two weeks and allow to dry, or else give your baby the essence orally. Emergency Essence applied topically is also very effective.

NAPPY RASH

Nappy rash usually happens when your baby has been wearing a wet nappy for too long. However, even when you are very careful about cleaning your baby's bottom and changing her nappies frequently, she may still develop nappy rash. The rash can become very inflamed and the skin may even blister. Always seek help from your health practitioner if you are concerned about the rash.

Nappy rash responds well to Emergency Essence, which can be used for any kind of rash. Either dab it onto the rash with a cotton wool ball, or spray it from a misting bottle and allow it to dry. Change your baby's nappy frequently, and use just plain water to clean the area. When it's possible, leave the nappy off so that the area is exposed to fresh air and has a better chance of healing quickly.

I am frequently told at workshops how effective Emergency Essence is in treating nappy rash. Parents tell me that as soon as their baby shows any sign of rash or chafing on their skin they apply Emergency Essence cream. They report how quickly it works and how the rash completely disappears, even bad bouts of it.

Rashes

My little boy, Finlay who is now 20 months old, had been having a hard time with teething, they were all coming up at once. He had his first bout of nappy rash. I mixed up a bottle of Green Essence with only water and sprayed his bottom before I put on his cream at every nappy change for two days. Plus I added Green Essence and Emergency Essence to his bath at night. By the third day the nappy rash was all gone. My husband is now using it on his rashes he gets up on the mines.

Sarah O'Brien, Western Australia

WEANING YOUR BABY

Your child will benefit greatly from being exclusively breastfed for the first six months of her life. If she is, she's unlikely to have problems with obesity and her immune system will be much stronger. If there is breastfeeding for at least two years the baby will be more emotionally secure. It is a good idea to continue to breastfeed for anything up to three years, if that's possible.

Put off introducing solid foods to your baby until she is at least six months old because her digestive system won't be mature enough to handle it before then. Begin with small amounts of food, and stay calm and relaxed as you feed her. It's important that mealtimes are not stressful for you or your child.

During the weaning period the remedy Bottlebrush, in Calm and Clear Essence, will be useful. It relates to the bond between mother and child, and it will help to break the pattern of breastfeeding without affecting the bond between you and your baby. You will find it easier to make that separation if you are also taking Bottlebrush yourself.

Successful weaning

I have successfully used Bottlebrush and Boronia (what I call the 'Moving On' drops) for helping people successfully stop smoking and also for helping mothers and toddlers during the weaning phase of breastfeeding (interesting linking breastfeeding and cigarette smoking!). I prescribe it twice a day for two weeks with an extra dose when breastfeeding is desired (and not forthcoming). The weaning process involves a pull between letting go of and 'pining for' with both the mother and the toddler. Many women I have given this mix to have found it helpful in reducing daytime feeds especially in cases where the feeding has become excessive and therefore unpleasant. However, the mother must be ready to begin the letting go process.

Barbara Murphy, Victoria, Australia

Guilty feelings

Sturt Desert Rose can be a very good remedy for you if you are feeling guilty about not letting your baby have the breast. It helps you have the courage to do what you have to do, even if your child is crying and very upset. Reassuring your child and giving her lots of love is most important at this time. It is a big step towards independence.

Ian

Projectile vomiting

A mother brought her ten-month-old baby boy to me because he was projectile vomiting during or just after eating. After hearing the mother's story, I prescribed for the baby:

- Dog Rose for fear;
- Five Corners for low self-esteem because his mother worried about his physical development;
- Paw Paw to help with digestion;
- Crowea, a good combination with Paw Paw for digestive disorders. It strengthens, calms and centres the body and mind.

The mother called three days later to say her son had not vomited since the second day on the essences and was smiling and laughing again.

Zdenka Dolejska, New South Wales, Australia

TEETHING PROBLEMS

Your baby's first teeth will start to come through when she is about six months old, although some babies teethe a little earlier than this and some later. She may grizzle because of the discomfort, and you may notice her cheek is red on the side where the tooth is breaking through. If your baby is uncomfortable and grizzling with teething pain, Emergency Essence will help her. It will ease the pain and also settle any fear, and give your baby the courage to deal with the pain and discomfort.

THE CHOICE OF CIRCUMCISION

Circumcision used to be performed routinely on newborn boys, but these days only about 10 per cent of male babies are circumcised. The main reason behind circumcision today would be for cultural and religious reasons as the current official medical point of view, especially in developed countries, is that there are no medical reasons for routine neonatal circumcision. Doctors who do advocate circumcision quote research that suggests circumcision can reduce the occurrence of urinary tract infections and decrease HIV infection in men, and even argue that it can reduce cervical cancer in female partners of circumcised men. There are also some uncommon medical conditions where circumcision is recommended and indicated.

There can be complications, although this applies to only about 3 per cent of cases. The main problems can be bleeding after the operation and infection, though both of these are usually dealt with quite successfully.

The issue can be very bewildering for parents. The remedy Paw Paw, which is in Cognis Essence, is great for parents to help them make a decision.

Circumcision
If your son is circumcised, use Emergency Essence together with Slender Rice Flower for a few days before and two weeks after the surgery, both topically and orally, to help heal the cut and avoid any scarring. Follow this procedure for any surgery.
Ian

VACCINATION

During this first year of your child's life you will need to make a decision about vaccinations. Parents want to do the best for their children but unfortunately it's not always easy to get the full story on vaccination.

Vaccines don't guarantee protection from disease, as they do not provide immunity to the disease. The only natural immunity to a disease or infection comes from getting that infection. Even those who have been vaccinated will at some point be susceptible to the illness they were originally vaccinated against. Parents often think their children are receiving pure vaccines, but whistleblowers within drug companies say it is very difficult to get a pure vaccine, that there are very often other viruses present. Some vaccines contain genetically engineered animal bacterial and viral DNA as well as yeast. There have been no long-term studies on this and nearly all studies on vaccination are paid for by the pharmaceutical companies making the vaccines.

Mercury is also in vaccines, and is a known neurotoxin. It is used as a preservative. The levels of mercury in vaccines are sometimes five times higher than what's recommended as a safe level. Other substances found in vaccines include formaldehyde and acelaldehyde, both very toxic ingredients. Most vaccines are basically a chemical cocktail.

Your child's immune system

The best way to boost your child's immune system is to breastfeed.

There has been a 1300 per cent increase in autism in Western countries over the last ten years, and a lot of evidence is pointing towards the correlation between vaccines and this rise in incidence. These days children are receiving far more vaccines than children of a generation ago. By the age of five or six, Australian children will have received about 50 vaccines, whereas fifteen years ago children of that same age would have received eighteen.

Ian

If you have looked at all the evidence and decided it's in your child's best interest for her to be vaccinated, I'd suggest giving her Emergency Essence for a few days immediately before and after the vaccination. Follow this with Purifying Essence taken for one month to help remove all neurotoxins and other chemicals found in the vaccines.

Important: Under no circumstances allow your child to be vaccinated if he is sick or has a fever, as there is a much greater likelihood of serious reactions if this occurs.

In Japan, the age for vaccinations has been put back to after one year of age, rather than at two months, four months and six months. By then children are neurologically much more advanced and can cope with these toxins somewhat better.

There is a strong theory that autism only developed as a result of vaccinations. In the United States in the 1920s when vaccination was introduced, it was not free: only rich people could afford vaccinations. In fact, autism at that point was referred to as the 'affluent disease' because it only struck in those areas where families had enough wealth to buy the vaccines. When vaccination became part of public health, widespread across socioeconomic groups, autism also spread across all these groups. There's been a great increase in autism, and today approximately one in 160 children is medically considered autistic. There are also concerns that the high levels of auto-immune diseases such as diabetes and asthma, and allergies in children, are the result of vaccinations. It's estimated that only 10 per cent of reactions to vaccinations are reported.

The live virus vaccines—for measles, mumps, rubella and chicken pox—can be carried in the body for three months after vaccination and can be transmitted to people who come in contact with the vaccinated person. The only cause of polio in Australia in the last 30 years, with the exception of imported cases from overseas, has been the actual polio vaccine itself. The remedy Jacaranda can help clear some of the side effects from the polio vaccine.

Whether to immunise

If you are unsure about whether to immunise your child, take Paw Paw, found in Cognis Essence, to help you make a decision. If you fear making the wrong decision Illawarra Flame Tree can help you, giving you the confidence to take responsibility.

Ian

If your child is already vaccinated

If your child is already vaccinated and this information worries you, then the metaphysical point of view may help. As mentioned earlier, children know exactly what is going to happen to them before they are incarnated: they choose their parents and family circumstances, so don't give yourself a hard time. To help counteract any neurotoxins or heavy metals your child might have absorbed from the vaccines, give Purifying Essence for a month.

Sometimes the vaccination, especially if there's a reaction, can affect the cranial bones in the skull. These are very soft bones that expand and contract as your child is breathing. In many children with learning problems, these cranial bones have become quite jammed up and rigid. Boab and Bush Fuchsia are remedies to help with this problem. Any child with rigidity in the cranial bones is far more likely to have problems with learning. Bush Fuchsia is specific, and in my opinion unsurpassed, for treating all learning problems.

ALLERGIES

In my work using iridology as a naturopath over the last 30 years, I've noticed that the older generations had greater physical strength then we do today. You only have to think of the pioneers who went to new areas, worked very hard to clear land and to create crops and so on to see how strong they were. But they had less emotional flexibility and what we see now is that, although children aren't as physically robust as their forebears, they have greater emotional flexibility. The pace of life has changed dramatically, and now new generations are a lot more in touch with their emotions.

However, with this greater sensitivity has come a greater susceptibility to allergies*. There are other factors, too: for example, it has been shown that vaccinations can increase the likelihood of allergic reactions. Children who haven't been breastfed are more likely to be allergic than children who were breastfed for at least six months.

One of the main remedies in helping with allergies is Fringed Violet, which will decrease your child's reactivity to the allergen. I combine this remedy with Dagger Hakea, which on the emotional level addresses resentment. If you are annoyed or irritated by someone and you do not resolve the issue, then you are more likely to internalise the problem and be easily irritated by your environment, whether it be the food you eat, the air you breathe or things that come into contact with your skin. Emergency Essence is very good for reducing an initial acute allergic reaction.

In the event of a severe allergic reaction (anaphylaxis), urgent and immediate medical treatment is required as this can be life-threatening. Anaphylaxis is characterised by the rapid increase of any of the following symptoms:

- deep flushing or cyanosis (a bluish tinge to the skin);
- severe coughing or wheezing;
- blurred vision;
- a weak or barely detectable pulse;
- loss of consciousness;
- vomiting; and/or
- shock.

Use Emergency Essence every few minutes until medical help arrives. If there is a lot of mucus being produced as part of the allergic response then Bush Iris is very helpful. There will be fewer allergies to food if the child is digesting their food very well. Paw Paw and Crowea in Calm and Clear Essence aid digestion.

Children are likely to have the same susceptibility to allergens as their parents, so this should be examined also. If there is a strong family allergic reaction, then think of giving Boab along with Emergency Essence.

Wang Yun Ting of Taiwan has successfully treated very allergic people by giving them Macrocarpa to build up their energy levels and help their immune systems. This remedy works on the adrenals, which are also affected by stress.

Allergies

I received a call from the mother of G who had been collected from school, where everything was giving her allergies, including the carpet. Her nose was stuffed up, her eyes were itchy and she wouldn't stop rubbing them. The doctor tried everything and was resorting to giving her weekly injections, which the mother didn't want. I prescribed Bush Iris, Dagger Hakea, Fringed Violet and Tall Mulla Mulla. She had two bottles of this and it worked very effectively. G and her family had, before I had treated them, moved back to Samoa but had to return as G was allergic to everything there.

Joy Andreadarkis, New South Wales, Australia

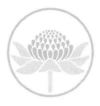

6

THE TODDLER YEARS

When your child is between one and three years of age she will become more competent and more mobile, and even more curious and communicative.

At this stage she will want her needs met immediately, and will let you know if she is unhappy. Gradually she will learn self-control, and this is partly due to the fact that she is developing language skills that allow her to communicate what it is she wants. Learning self-control is part of the socialisation process, and your child needs you to set boundaries in a reasonable and consistent way so that she learns what behaviour is acceptable and what isn't.

As she grows and develops your child will inevitably face physical and emotional challenges, and she will feel particularly secure if she senses that you are confident in dealing with them. One of the great aspects of Bush Essences is that they are a safe tool that helps a child and empowers the parents to deal with their children's challenges. When you are calm and unruffled, your child is more likely to feel secure and comfortable. This in itself is a good start in addressing any challenges that might arise.

THE VALUE OF PLAY

Until they are three years old children will usually play on their own, even when they are in the company of other children. But around the age of three they will play together with other children for longer and longer periods. They start learning how to work out differences, and the more they play with each other the more complex their games start to become.

The value of play can never be underestimated in the healthy development of children. It's through play that they learn about the world and build their social skills. Their fantasy play allows them to imagine new possibilities, and this is the best possible preparation for life. All the well-known and respected educationalists, such as Rudolf Steiner, believed that children must have time for imaginative and creative play. Expose your child to music, fairytales and games, and avoid giving too many directions. The point of play is that it is free and unstructured. Children generally won't need much help to play, though Little Flannel Flower will assist and Turkey Bush will enhance creativity.

TANTRUMS

Most children will have tantrums*, and they usually start at around eighteen months of age. Before that they may experience pre-toddler mood swings. The main difference between the two is that tantrums are more intense and there's a greater degree of confrontation, especially with parents.

There is great variation between children and their tantrums. In a younger child, a tantrum could be due to frustration or to the fact that he can't tell you what he feels or wants. He may be irritated that he can't do things like dress himself. Then there's the anger and frustration of not getting what he wants when he wants it, or of not being able to control what's happening around him. Another cause of tantrums is the child's limited understanding of the world, which can lead to fear and confusion, which in turn can lead to a tantrum. You can use either Emergency Essence or Confid Essence to help with fear as well as talking to and reassuring the child.

For a little child the intensity of his emotions can be quite scary. Sometimes he has so much energy building up that he has to find a way to release that energy. Sometimes after a tantrum he may become very needy and clingy and you'll need to show plenty of love at these times, giving him hugs and reassurance that you love him.

One of the most important things you can do for the emotional development of your child is to help him learn he can't always get what he wants when he wants it. And for your child's own safety, he needs to know that there are limits. You have to take charge. An extreme example here is if your child wants to run across the street without any adult to supervise him or to keep him safe: just as in this example, your young child needs to learn that you are doing the best for him by keeping him safe.

Children of the new generation
Children born from the late 1990s onwards want more explained to them; they want to know what is going on. If you explain what and why things are being done, you may be able to short circuit a tantrum so that it doesn't happen at all.
Ian

It's wise to prepare ahead of time to avoid temper tantrums in little ones. If you know that a stressful situation is coming up, such as shopping or going for a long car ride, make sure your child is well rested and well fed and take snacks along. If you're going on a longer trip, once you've arrived allow your child to run around a bit to use up some of his pent-up energy.

If you are at home when a tantrum occurs, put your child in his room and tell him not to come out until he is in a calmer state. Place him there firmly, shut the door and move away. If the tantrum is in public, it's best to remove your child from that situation and find somewhere that is private and quiet.

Tantrums

For weeks Tim had been extremely difficult to please, grouchy, tantrums at the drop of a hat, sometimes three or four a day, tired, naughty etc. All my usual behavioural techniques were useless and he was really wearing me down. After working with Mountain Devil he was much happier and easier to live with. The change in his behaviour was a very pleasant surprise.
Jenny Hill, New South Wales, Australia

Either Emergency Essence or Calm and Clear Essence will help to settle your child, addressing that sense of losing control. Spray the mist around him and you'll see the difference.

Calming tantrums

Bess is a five-year-old girl who had been having tantrums for about six months—big ones that could last anywhere between ten minutes and two to three hours, with yelling, kicking and screaming. I made up a remedy for her with Dagger Hakea to help her with her attitude toward her parents and siblings, as she was saying how much she hated them, and becoming embarrassed afterwards but unable to say sorry for her behaviour. I gave her Dog Rose of the Wild Forces to help her gain control of her emotions, Fringed Violet for protection and Mountain Devil for the unconditional love that she needed to embrace.

After four days she had only had one tantrum and declared that the drops weren't working. But she said she felt different, though she wasn't sure how. After two weeks the tantrums were almost non-existent and, more importantly, she felt different about them and the need to have them. A month later she had not had any major tantrums.

Now when the tantrums are mentioned, she puts on a wry smile and makes no comment. A definite success story!

Lisa Higgins, New South Wales, Australia

Around three to four years of age there can often be battles of will when children will defy their parents' authority. By the end of this stage a child will come to realise they can't get everything they want and they have to consider other people and their needs. If, however, they are still overly focused on their own needs by this age then I recommend giving Kangaroo Paw.

Balanced discipline

Be aware of whether you are over-disciplining your child. When there are too many rules and regulations, young children can react with temper tantrums. You don't have to have a battle over every issue.

The remedy Yellow Cowslip Orchid is useful, especially for men, when there's an insistence on things having to be done a certain way and frustration when the small child doesn't obey. But it's always best to give your child praise and acknowledgment and to encourage the good things he is doing. It is important not to focus on criticism or draw attention to what you are not happy with.

Setting boundaries
Consistency is essential. If you tell your child what needs to happen, stick to it and avoid giving in. Taking Flannel Flower will help you set strong boundaries.
Ian

Smacking is not the way to teach your child good behaviour. In fact, smacking models bad behaviour; imagine smacking your child while saying 'Don't smack other children'. Young children have little self-control, and they learn gradually to manage their emotions by watching how their parents react to life. Praise, encouragement and love will guide your child towards the right way to behave.

All the same, it is the nature of toddlers to have tantrums. They are trying to establish some independence and they protest when they're told they can't do something. It's important for you to remain calm, so when your child does have a tantrum Emergency Essence will help you. The remedy Dog Rose of the Wild Forces in Emergency Essence is useful for you if you feel you are losing control along with your child. Arguing with your child or becoming angry will only make matters worse.

Also acknowledge your child's feelings. Say that you know he is really upset and frustrated so that he has a sense of being understood. Ask him if he'd like a cuddle. Many children respond well to this approach.

After the tantrum

After a tantrum, when your child has settled down, talk to him, let him know you are not happy about what happened, and also give him a hug and reassure him that he is still loved regardless of his behaviour. As your child gets a little older, you could discuss with him other ways to deal with frustration, such as drawing how he is feeling rather than having a tantrum.

Ian

Aggressive, clingy behaviour

A mother brought her little boy to me because his behaviour was aggressive, mainly towards her. He was very demanding and moody. He'd witnessed physical abuse by his father towards his mother, before they'd separated. Tantrums were fairly frequent occurrences. He'd often wake through the night crying, often wet and hard to settle back down. He'd also had a traumatic birth and his first twelve months were chaotic. I prescribed several essences, including:

- Fringed Violet to repair his aura, damaged by his traumatic birth;
- Kangaroo Paw to address how he treated his mother; and
- Dog Rose to alleviate his fears.

After two weeks of taking the essences morning and night, a big change was evident in the boy. His grandmother asked me what miracle drops I'd given her grandson. He was less clingy, anxious, more agreeable and his sleeping was more settled.

Sheree Ashurst, Queensland, Australia

FRUSTRATION BEFORE A NEW STAGE

Child professionals have noted that some children will have tantrums in the lead-up to a major stage of development, such as crawling or walking—she is almost there but hasn't quite mastered the skill yet and therefore reacts with frustration.

Purifying Essence will help a child who is frustrated as she approaches a new stage of development. One of its remedies, Wild Potato Bush, will address frustration, and another, Bauhinia, will help her be more open to change, especially if the frustration is due to holding back because she feels insecure.

Mother Kim Mann reports that when her daughter Charlotte began trying to crawl at six months she would become frustrated with her lack of progress. 'A dose of Wild Potato Bush for a two-week period helped her move through this time with less frustration,' says Kim. 'I also used it when she began to show signs of moving around the furniture and getting to her feet at about nine months. She is currently finishing another course as she starts to make the transition to walking on her own and it is helping her yet again!'

STARTING ON TOILET TRAINING

Success with toilet training depends on your child's neurological development which, with the exception of using Bush Fuchsia, can't be forced or sped up. By the age of two, most children start to have some voluntary control and are ready for toilet training. Until this age, food and drink stimulate contractions which lead to a bowel movement or urination after meals.

Preparing for toilet training
The remedy Bush Fuchsia, in Cognis Essence, can promote neurological development so that children are ready for toilet training.
Ian

Young children can't tell the difference between when they are wet or dry, or when their nappy is soiled. When children do start to recognise the difference between wet and dry, they do not like the sensation of being wet. By two and a half years of age, the majority of children will be dry most of the time. Some children will have control over their bladder first, while others will have control over their bowels first.

It's a good idea for you to explain to your child what toilet training is all about. Children today need things explained to them rather than being told, even when the issue is toilet training. By giving clear explanations so that they understand why they are going to be toilet trained, you can save a lot of time and drama. Once your child knows why, he is more likely to follow and take on the new learning.

Bedwetting

I got wonderful results with Dog Rose for my boy of six who was still bedwetting three to four times a week. When I started Dog Rose he was wet every night—now he has been dry for one month.

Christiane Hougardy, Belgium

If your child is starting bowel training, you could give him Bottlebrush, which is in both Calm and Clear Essence and Purifying Essence, to help him let go of old routines and the pattern of using nappies. A good technique is to get your child to sit on the potty for up to about five minutes on waking in the morning and in the afternoons. If your child 'produces', then give lots of acknowledgment and praise. For a child who has trouble sitting still for a number of minutes—and that's most toddlers!—Calm and Clear Essence will help.

When your child has woken with a dry nappy over a number of nights, you can start to leave the nappy off at night. The usual time for children to be night trained is just before their third birthday, though each child is individual.

By age five there are still quite a lot of children bedwetting, normally about 10 per cent. This is most likely to occur if one or especially both parents had problems in this area. The main remedies for bedwetting are Dog Rose, which works on the kidneys and bladder, while if there was a family pattern then add Boab. I've found a fantastic combination to treat bedwetting is Red Helmet Orchid together with Dog Rose. In Chinese medicine the kidneys and bladder represent fear and it has been found that if there is some anxiety or fear, especially in the home environment, it is more likely associated with the father, probably as fathers are physically bigger, have a louder voice and can often take on a stern, disciplinary role.

Nightmares and bedwetting

A four-year-old boy who wet his bed was brought to me. He wet his bed almost every night. He had a well-developed imagination and also had regular nightmares about monsters etc. His father was a nice man, but tended to be an authoritative parent believing that a child should not be encouraged to give in to his fears. I gave Dog Rose for the boy's fears and kidney problems and bedwetting in general; Red Helmet Orchid just in case he had unresolved father issues; Boab, as the little boy was turning out so much like his father that his family had taken to calling him Ditto; and Grey Spider Flower for his nightmares. Ethan still wet the bed the first night but then he didn't wet the bed for the whole of the fortnight while on the essences. He wet the bed after three days off the essences and now only occasionally bed wets. Six weeks later Ethan is now getting up in the middle of the night and going to the toilet by himself, something he'd been too afraid to do before.

Anne Robinson, Queensland, Australia

As children get older, around the age of seven, and are wanting to socialise more and have more sleepovers, bedwetting can have a huge impact on them. They will quite often become shy and self-conscious about their bedwetting and will not want to attend sleepovers. It can affect their self-esteem, so Confid Essence or Billy Goat Plum may be used for shame and embarrassment.

Bedwetting

I successfully treated a little girl, Amy, for bedwetting. She is now not wetting her bed and tells her mother to please not come and get her up in the night to go to the toilet, she is not afraid now and can't see the scary heads of the people any more in the room. She now doesn't need to get up until 7 o'clock in the morning. When she was little she had received a bad kick between her legs and ever since then had bladder infections on and off. The essences have cleared the infections as well. Her mum told me that when she takes her drops she prays with the bottle first and then takes them, and she told her mother that at first she asked the flowers to help her to not be afraid at night and take away the heads of the scary people around the bed. Now that she doesn't see those scary heads her mum said she just prays in silence and takes her drops. I wonder what she is saying to the flowers now!

Marg Kehoe, Peru

CONSTIPATION

If your child is constipated a bowel movement can be painful, so make sure you give your child plenty of liquids. A lot of young children today are drawn to more liquid, juices in particular, and this is good for nourishment. Water is also important to help them move their bowels more frequently. If they are anxious, give Emergency Essence to help relax them.

Bottlebrush is the remedy for constipation*. Adults have commented that while taking Bottlebrush they felt as though a bottlebrush was literally put up inside them to clean them out! It is a very effective remedy.

Ideally, your child's bowels will open three times a day. I've had parents come to me worried about their children going so often, but be assured that provided the stool is not too loose, as in diarrhoea, then a three-times-a-day habit it is a very healthy thing. Once a day is a minimum.

Extreme constipation

A five-year-old girl was brought to me. She had suffered extreme constipation ever since she started solid food at six months. She had just started school and was having problems adjusting. She had been on a laxative since she was twelve months old and because going to the toilet hurt her and she was now scared of going, she ate and drank little, which only made the problem worse. I gave her Purifying Essence which contained:

- Bauhinia to work on the ileocaecal valve and to help shift her reluctance to change her ways to resolve the constipation;
- Bottlebrush to act on the large intestine and to help clear out old waste. It would also help with the major life change of going to school and with letting go;
- Dog Rose for the fear and to help the kidneys; and
- Bush Iris to work on the lymphatics to cleanse and purify.

The essences worked within two days and within four weeks the problem was totally resolved. She had stopped all laxatives and was not frightened about eating or drinking. I was ecstatic and her parents were elated their daughter wasn't suffering as it had been a never-ending worry for them for five years.

Simone McCallum, Queensland, Australia

RASHES

Skin rashes* are a sign of toxic waste building up internally that has not been correctly eliminated through the lymphatic system or other organs of elimination—kidney, bowel, liver. If a child is taken to a medical doctor with eczema, the common treatment is a cortisone-based cream. The effect of this is that the elimination through the skin is suppressed but later on, at about age three to five, these children commonly develop asthma.

From the naturopathic point of view, it is much better to allow your child to eliminate and to work with Purifying Essence so the rash is not severe. Give it to your child for up to a month. It works on all the organs of elimination—kidney, liver, bowel and lymphatics—to help with detoxification. Topically, use Green Essence in a misting bottle morning and night; spray on the affected area and allow to dry.

Lead poisoning

A one-year-old boy was diagnosed with high levels of lead poisoning (24 points, with 4 points being normal), so I prescribed a bottle of Purifying Essence. The nurse was 'totally amazed' that his lead levels dropped 8 points in just a month. Lead blood levels usually drop only a few points every few months. His mother was breastfeeding, and she is taking the essences to protect her second baby.

Arlene Riddick, United States

RISING TEMPERATURE

Children have a very strong, vital force and if there is something wrong in their body they tend to burn it up quickly. This is why children experience many more fevers* than adults do. When a small one has a temperature it is not a catastrophe, it's basically the child releasing toxins from the body, and with love and positive energy this will be successfully done.

Temperature

I use Mulla Mulla automatically when my children have a temperature. It helps them rest and allows their bodies to deal with and fight infection. I'm also amazed at the instant effects on burns.

Janne Ferguson, Victoria, Australia

Children have the ability to reset their thermostat for fevers up to about 41 degrees. Paracetamol is a liver toxin and the most common cause of drug overdose in children. If you choose to give it to your child ensure you follow the dosage guidelines, particularly in regard to your child's age. A study published in *The Lancet* in 2008 reported that there is an association with an increased risk of asthma, eczema and allergic runny nose later in childhood if acetaminophen (which is sold worldwide under brand names such as Panadol and Tylenol, and is an ingredient in many other pain relievers) is used in the first year of a child's life.

The Bush Essence for fevers is Mulla Mulla, which eases the distress children can feel about the burning sensation as well as helping to safely manage the fever.

To help ease the fever, you could also make a lemon compress for your child's feet. Cut the lemon under water, put the pieces into socks that have been soaked in water and place them on her feet. Cover with dry socks and rest her feet on a hot water bottle.

From the metaphysical point of view, the most important thing you can do when your child has a fever is to give her lots of love, to hold her, put your arms around her, and reassure her. Don't put a child with a fever in a room on her own, but keep her in contact with you.

Another common cause of fevers for young children is teething. Often their faces can be flushed where the tooth or teeth are coming through. Emergency Essence is excellent to help them with any irritability and grumpiness and to alleviate the pain and discomfort they are experiencing. You can give it as often as every ten to fifteen minutes. Some parents have said that putting drops of Emergency Essence on a moist piece of cloth that the child chews on settles them. For the fever, again use Mulla Mulla or the combination Solaris Essence that it is in. You can give it quite frequently if the fever is high (every 15 minutes) until it comes down and the child is more settled, or every hour or so if it is not as severe.

Rather than relying on the temperature alone to gauge your child's health, check on how your child is feeling. If your child is irritable and can't be consoled, seek medical advice. A red, flushed appearance is a normal response to fever, but a green or grey colour in the face indicates something else. In this case, get medical advice.

Important: Avoiding dehydration

Especially if your child has a fever, check that she remains hydrated. Your child is NOT dehydrated if:

- she cries with tears;
- the inside of her mouth is wet; and/or
- she urinates twice in 24 hours.

If you are concerned about your child's hydration levels, place 7 drops of She Oak in water and give it every ten minutes or so until your child is rehydrated.

If her eyes appear at all sunken, take your child to a hospital straight away.

If your child fits

Sometimes a child will have a fit when he has a high temperature. This is known as a febrile convulsion, and is not uncommon.

Febrile convulsions most commonly occur between six months and three years of age and rarely occur after five years of age. About 5 per cent of children will have a febrile convulsion. If your child has one, he may become either stiff or floppy, jerk and twitch or have difficulty breathing. Seek immediate medical attention if your child convulses. If your child has one fit then he is likely to have another (that is, he is susceptible to fits), but working with Mulla Mulla can often reduce this likelihood; it is in Solaris Essence. The fit can come on very quickly, so give Mulla Mulla at the first sign of fever.

Dealing with trauma

As a parent you can benefit from taking Emergency Essence to help you deal with the trauma of watching your child experience a febrile convulsion. It is particularly important for you to remain calm, and Emergency Essence will certainly help.

Convulsions

If your child starts fitting, put a few drops of Emergency Essence on his head. Place him on his side so that it is easier for his airway to stay open. Any difficulty in breathing is usually due to a tightening of the bronchials, and Crowea, in Emergency Essence, will help relax them.
Ian

HELPING YOUR CHILD SLEEP

Children's diets can affect their sleeping habits and can sometimes lead to sleeping problems*. Foods containing preservatives and lots of sugar, especially if eaten just before bedtime, can keep them more active and less likely to sleep. Take a close look at what your child is eating, particularly before bedtime, if they are having trouble sleeping.

Explain to your child why it is important to get sleep. You could give 'warning times', showing him on the clock that he has fifteen minutes before he is expected to be in bed.

One of the most effective things you can do to promote sleep is to create a calm environment around your child at bedtime. Spraying Calm and Clear Essence is very beneficial, especially in his bedroom. You can also pat some onto his hands and face at night as well as giving the drops. In Calm and Clear Essence are remedies that help release muscles and help a child who is always on the go to quieten down. It brings them back into their body and slows them down. Little children are very sensitive and easily stimulated. Calm and Clear Essence will also help them tune inwards and go off to sleep more quickly. If there is anything bothering them, it helps them to stop worrying about it.

Natural sleep rhythms

Ben's parents reported that he just wouldn't go to bed at night. He was prescribed Bush Fuchsia, which was added to Emergency Essence, to help him get back into natural rhythms. It worked within days, and the only downside for Ben's parents

79

was that his body's natural rhythm is to wake at sunrise. This meant no more sleeping in for them!
Ian

Regular routines are important for children. Make sure that in the period leading up to bedtime there is no wild activity and that your child is starting to slow down. It's a good time for quietly reading stories.

Lack of sleep

If you are feeling frazzled, tired or impatient because your child is not sleeping, your state can flow on to your child, making matters even worse. Calm and Clear Essence will help here. Lack of sleep can create a lot of distress and sometimes parents can become short tempered and even aggressive. Dog Rose of the Wild Forces, which is in Emergency Essence, is the remedy if there is that tendency to lose control.

If both you and your partner become stressed because of a lack of sleep, one in particular may feel unsupported and constantly tired. You no longer have close, intimate time together because your child is in your bed or you are up attending to your child all night. Relationship Essence can be good here, especially if there is resentment between you and your partner.

Sleep deprivation
For sleep deprivation over a long period of time, Dynamis Essence will help you overcome exhaustion and weariness.
Ian

Children's disrupted sleep patterns

Some children can have difficulty adjusting when daytime naps are tapering off. If your child is not sleeping well at night it could be that she is sleeping too long during the day, and the answer may be to cut the naps back or to eliminate them altogether. Your child might be a bit more tired and grumpy during the day, but she will go to bed earlier and have better quality sleep. What's more, parents will have the opportunity for more time with each other.

Some children who used to have good sleep patterns may start waking in the middle of the night. It may be due to an illness or an upset. Take a good look at what is happening in your child's environment and give the appropriate remedy. It may be that you have moved house, or there is a new baby in the family, for example. Disrupted night sleeping may also stem from illness, or there might be some upsets in the home or a death in the family. Give Red Suva Frangipani for family upsets, and Sturt Desert Pea for grief. If there has been a change of house or a new sibling has arrived then essences such as Bottlebrush could be used.

Waking in the night may go on for a few nights, but if it continues any longer a habit can start to develop. Give Bottlebrush to help break a new habit. If your child regularly wakes during the night, look into various techniques such as controlled crying and sleep training. Any technique will work much more effectively if you use essences as well, especially if you spray Calm and Clear Essence or Emergency Essence.

Something else to consider is that if children are very sensitive they can pick up on energies present in the room. Who was living in the house before you were? Maybe the energy relates to people who have visited. It could even be that lots of arguments have gone on in bedrooms between people who previously lived in the house. Children may also pick up on what we would call ghosts or lost souls hovering around. Space Clearing Essence is very useful, especially if your child is usually quite settled but is disturbed or anxious being in her bedroom.

For parents: Letting your child cry

Take Emergency Essence for yourself if you become upset at having to let your child cry for a short time on his own.

Ian

Night terrors

While nightmares usually occur in children over three years of age, younger children are more likely to experience night terrors. These are when a child wakes in a great state of terror and is oblivious to her surroundings or her parents' attempts to calm and soothe her. This can last for up to 20 or 30 minutes.

It can be terrifying seeing your child react in this way, but getting angry, shaking her or trying other ways to bring her back to consciousness won't work. Emergency Essence will help you sit calmly and quietly, reassuring her during the episode. Surprisingly, children rarely remember anything of the night terror the next morning.

Nightmares

Nightmares* can be terrifying for children. Your child might wake from a nightmare feeling very distressed and cry for you. Hold her and reassure her so that she feels safe. Give her Emergency Essence, which is excellent for nightmares, because it contains Grey Spider Flower for terror as well as Dog Rose of the Wild Forces for extreme fear.

Nightmares may be associated with past times, because young children process a great deal of their former lives during their early years, especially their most recent life. For many of them it can be traumatic. Green Spider Orchid is the remedy for nightmares and phobias from past life experiences and it can be added to Emergency Essence if the nightmares are frequent.

I also suggest playing the White Light CD at night, before bedtime, because it is very calming for children. Sound (pure vibration) is a force inherent in all things. It has a powerful effect on the cellular structure of human bodies and a very profound influence on the psyche and soul. My wife, harpist Jane Rosenson, and violinist Kirsten Williams, both exceptional musicians, have recorded the beautiful White Light CD, which contains excerpts from eight musical masterpieces. Listening to this uplifting CD will help bring you into balance.

Problems going to bed

There can be a number of reasons for problems that occur at bedtime. There can be separation anxiety, for which Illawarra Flame Tree is a good remedy. Some children enjoy being around their family, so may procrastinate by continually asking for drinks or one more story. Give them reassurance that they are loved, that you will be there in the morning and be firm when you put out the light. Calm and Clear drops can help them to settle down in this situation. Young children are very sensitive so they are easily stimulated; Calm and Clear will help them relax and go to sleep more quickly.

Nightmares

I gave my daughter Fringed Violet, Green Spider Orchid, Grey Spider Flower and sprayed her bedroom with Space Clearing Essence, all of which had been recommended by the Bush Essence office because my daughter had been frightened at night by witches, monsters etc. This morning she told me she had a dream about the ugly old witch again but in this dream the witch was really nice and friendly, not scary at all. Even though others were scared of her my daughter was not, she actually liked the witch a lot.

Kelley Colyer, New South Wales, Australia

A lot of young children are susceptible to energies. They are very psychic, and they may see some unpleasant energies in the room. Ask your child what it is she is seeing. If she is fearful of seeing things, sit with her and pray together to the angels and God to provide extra protection. Creating an energy field together in this way can be powerfully reassuring for a child. You might be surprised at what your child sees and what she tells you about, and what you're able to create together.

Disturbed sleep

A girl who suffered epilepsy was having disturbed sleep and nightmares. There was some aggressive behaviour with screaming bouts, and she would wet the bed at night. I gave her Grey Spider Flower and within a week she was sleeping much better and was now dry at night. The screaming had stopped too.

Vera, United Kingdom

TROUBLE COMMUNICATING

Toddlers often become frustrated that they can't yet communicate what they want. This can be the case especially for boys, whose language develops later than for girls, and often they will react to the frustration by having a tantrum.

Difficulty communicating

My little boy was having trouble telling me what he wanted, and I noticed he was becoming more and more withdrawn. I gave him Flannel Flower to help him with his communication, and I followed that with Confid Essence to boost his self-confidence. He was so much happier and outgoing, and having a go at more words than before.

Christine Norley, South Australia

Stuttering

My son's vocabulary was always very advanced and when he was two and a half everyone commented on how well he spoke. A few months later he started stuttering. It happened overnight and was very severe. His first course of Bush Fuchsia provided immense relief. He was still in the severe category but there was a huge improvement. I continued with this essence and then added Paw Paw. After this he recorded his lowest stuttering rate ever at the clinic. He continued to show improvement in his speech, and now his stutter is barely noticeable.

Jenny Hill, New South Wales, Australia

It's important to let your child know you are listening to him, because it lets him know that you care about him and what he wants to tell you. Even when he does start to talk let him finish what he's saying, even if it takes some time. Don't hurry him along, but listen patiently. Gradually he'll have the language to communicate more clearly. The essence for clear communication is Flannel Flower, which also addresses openness and the expression of feelings. Give it to your child to help him communicate his wants and needs more clearly.

BITING AND HITTING OTHER CHILDREN

Small children can engage in behaviour that embarrasses their parents, and nothing much seems to stop it. An example is offered by Clare, whose young son Toby would often bite or hit other children at playgroup for no apparent reason. 'I felt like a bad mother,' she said. 'The other mothers were protective of their children, naturally, and Toby just wouldn't listen to me.' Toby was prescribed Mountain Devil, the main remedy for aggressive behaviour, and within days he was relaxed at playgroup and would play happily without attacking the other children.

Inconsolable

My toddler grandchild woke from a nap whining and unable to be consoled by anyone, including her mother. After three hours of listening to this, the entire household was on edge. I gave her mother a brief, simple description of how the essences work, and assured her they would not harm the child. The toddler would not take any drops under her tongue, so we applied seven drops of Emergency Essence to the crown of her head. Her reaction was to immediately put her hand on her head and then in her mouth. Within half an hour she had stopped whining and was smiling and talking happily. The effect was astounding. Her mum went home with a bottle of Emergency Essence.

Olwen Anderson, New South Wales, Australia

FEAR OF OTHERS

If your child seems to shrink back from strangers or have any fear of others*, it could be that he is very selective. Perhaps he can read auras, and because some people don't have good energy your child sees this and reacts to it. It could be that the 'stranger' has been angry, about being in a traffic jam, for example, and your child sees their aura and feels more anxious. Fringed Violet, in Emergency Essence, can be good for a child who is very sensitive. It helps him not pick up so much, and encloses him in a psychic 'bubble' if there are people around him who are upset.

Children of this generation are especially psychic and intuitive. There could be, energetically speaking, something about a person they don't like. Someone may appear friendly but if underneath they are a very angry person then that can appear in their aura and that's what a child will respond to. Sometimes a child's response is well founded and can prove a good protective mechanism; if a child only shrinks back from certain people, this is the key. He may be sensing something energetically: for example, such people may be rushed, or impatient, or may not like children.

Another reason for a child being fearful of others is that his mother might have suffered a lot of stress during the pregnancy, and a child picking up on these stress hormones can be more anxious than other children.

If your child is quite shy or fearful, then you can work with Dog Rose. This remedy is found in Confid Essence, and as your child's self-confidence increases he will be less likely to perceive people around him as threatening.

For parents: Fighting
If you and your partner argue, the remedy Dagger Hakea can help you let go of old resentments and grudges that keep coming back every time there is an argument. Mountain Devil and Black-eyed Susan will also help give you more tolerance and patience, and help you to be more forgiving.
Ian

EASILY UPSET

Children who are very sensitive can be easily upset. They pick up vibrations of people and situations very strongly. The more 2s your child has in their birth date, the greater their sensitivity.

Separation anxiety* could be affecting your child if she is easily upset, or a food intolerance* may also be affecting her.

Finding confidence

Toby started to become very clingy, following me around and crying unless I held him. I found Confid Essence worked wonders. In a short time he was more confident and would play happily without chasing me around.
Sharon, address withheld

THE ANXIOUS CHILD

Some children seem to suffer anxiety* much of the time. If this is the case with your child, consider what was going on for you and your partner when your child was in the womb, as well as the actual birth experience. If there was trauma, your child would have been directly affected by any stress hormones released in the mother's body. This may make your child hypervigilant, always on guard with a feeling she is not safe. She may also have trouble sleeping.

Clearing negative energy
Spraying the environment where your child plays and sleeps with Space Clearing Essence will clear any negative energy and create a harmonious environment.
Ian

A child will also be anxious and hypervigilant if she is raised in a family where there is any alcoholism or domestic violence, for example. It is estimated that around 5 per cent of the Australian population is alcoholic, and this has a direct effect on children. They can become anxious because they feel out of control, unsure of what might happen next. The remedy for a hypervigilant child is Hibbertia, though you should also consider using Emergency Essence first for anywhere from two to four weeks, to address the original trauma. If you know of the specific incident that you believe was the catalyst then address it with the relevant Bush Essence.

Birth trauma

The birth of Maree's daughter was very traumatic, and the baby was placed in a humidicrib afterwards. Maree's practitioner suggested this was behind the girl's behaviour when, at two years of age, Jessie was constantly anxious and no amount of reassurance was helping her. She was prescribed Fringed Violet, in Emergency Essence, to clear the trauma of her birth and the separation afterwards. Within days she was happier and far more settled than ever before.
Ian

Childcare and separation anxiety

For young children, being left with a babysitter or going to daycare or preschool and watching their parents leave can trigger separation anxiety*. For most children, separation anxiety begins at around six months of age and peaks at their first birthday. It tends to decrease by the age of three, but some children continue to suffer from it.

Separation Anxiety

Todd, a three-year-old, was becoming very clingy to his mother as time came for him to go to preschool. I made up a mixture of Crowea to calm his worries, Dog Rose for anxiety and Dog Rose of the Wild Forces to clear away the panic and terror. After taking this remedy for a week (7 drops morning and night) Todd started to become happier and more independent. When the time came for him to start preschool he was happy and confident and is now enjoying life to the full.

Jill Ramsden, United Kingdom

Generally speaking, boys tend to experience greater separation anxiety than girls, although certainly some girls will suffer from it. During the early years of one to three years of age, the child's stronger bond is with the mother. After that, the father's role becomes particularly important. Strengthening the bonding between mother and child will help him feel more confident and secure in himself. Bottlebrush is the remedy here, both for mother and child. It may seem a paradox, but Bottlebrush also helps with letting go, so it is beneficial when a child is a bit clingy.

Emergency Essence will help a child who becomes distressed at the separation. If your child is very distressed, it's a good idea to find someone close to him—a relative or close friend, for example, rather than a stranger—to take care of him, or to leave any separation for a few weeks or months if possible. Continue to give Bottlebrush so that the mother–child bond becomes very strong, because the more secure a child feels the easier he will find separation.

Routines

Because little children feel safer with an uninterrupted routine, make sure that the babysitter you employ keeps things as close to usual routine as possible while they are caring for your child.

Ian

Anxiety about school

A young girl in grade 3 was referred by the school's psychologist. She was missing up to two days a week of school and complaining of stomach problems, mainly to avoid school. She would become very distressed when her mother left her at school. She didn't live with her father, who yelled at her a lot. She always worried and it created a churning in her stomach, and would stop her going to sleep. If her mother yelled at her for doing something wrong she felt like she'd been punched in the stomach. If her mother was late picking her up from school she would worry there had been an accident or that her mother had forgotten and was not coming to pick her up. The Insight Card she chose, Crowea, is *the* remedy for worry. After just one week Jessie reported having attended six consecutive school days without any tears or anxiety, she was feeling positive about her teacher and not feeling sick before school. Crowea kept working well and in the next session she chose Dog Rose from the Insight Cards, the remedy for fear. Prior to that session she was still getting nervous but felt that she was worrying less. After six weeks I had a call from the school who were amazed at the transition of this little girl who now came so happily to school and managed to achieve a 100 per cent attendance record.

Janne Ferguson, Victoria, Australia

MANIPULATIVE BEHAVIOUR

Children can learn to use manipulative behaviour very early. They see that behaving in particular ways will result in certain responses from the people around them. This usually occurs because they want love and affection, and the remedy Rough Bluebell will help them let go of the manipulative behaviour so they can receive that love without playing games.

LEARNING TO SHARE

Very young children often need to be encouraged to share with others. They can become possessive about their toys, for example, and find it difficult to see other children play with them. You'll hear the word 'mine' said over and over, but this is usually a relatively short-lived stage. The remedy Bluebell will help even very young children to feel more comfortable about sharing.

Sometimes, though, the problem persists. It could be that in a past life a child has experienced a lack of food, water or air, and this time around they believe on a subconscious level there is not enough to go around. They feel driven to hold on to what they've got and not let others near it for fear of losing it. Bluebell will help them understand that there is plenty. Sometimes they can be this way not just with physical things but also with emotions; they only give out a little bit, fearful that if they give too much they'll run out.

As they get older this can cause real difficulties. If they feel there is only so much love they can give, they'll limit the amount of happiness they give to others and how much they receive themselves. Bluebell will address this tendency to hold back with loving.

Attachment to possessions

The remedy Bush Iris will help children who are very materialistic and/or are overly attached to their possessions and won't share them.
Ian

Some children can become very set in their ways and more stubborn, especially if there is an element of autism. These children like routine and access to a toy exactly when they want it, which can obviously mean they have difficulty sharing. Bluebell would still be used for aiding generosity and opening the heart but in this case I recommend you add it with Yellow Cowslip Orchid, to address the need to have everything in the exact same regimen.

For parents: Difficulty sharing

It can be difficult for parents to recognise that they themselves have trouble sharing with others. If you do see this aspect in yourself, then taking the remedy Boab will help break those generational patterns early on.
Ian

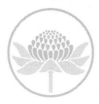

7

YOUR CHILD'S SPIRIT

Since the early 1980s until the end of the 1990s we witnessed a very different generation of children being born. The 'bridging generation' is one term that has been used to describe them. There is a marked shift in the qualities of these children compared to previous generations going back hundreds of years when there was a stong intellectual emphasis. Since the invention of the printing press, a fascination with and a movement towards intellectual knowledge has shaped humanity. At that time education shifted towards learning from books, and learning became more focused on interactions between people rather than interactions directly with the Earth, Nature and the wider world.

As Jan Thomas states in her book, *Chiron . . . On Children*: 'When books came the scholars taught what could be found in the books written by man and they lost the ability to read the "book of the heavens" and "the book of the earth". They also lost the ability to open their eyes and see the wonders that were around them in reality.' Very importantly, humankind's search for greater wisdom and knowledge of the mind led to a closing down of what is known as the feeling centre—an empathy for one another, and an empathy for the Earth and Nature. These new children are returning to and claiming this lost heritage.

It is interesting that all the children born since the year 2000 all have the number 2 in their birth date. In numerology, this number represents intuition, sensitivity and cooperation. Another aspect that is very marked with so many, but not all, children born in this millennium is their tremendous capacity for love. This is one of their great gifts they bring down: the ability to heal others through their loving natures. Many of the babies of this new millennium are, even straight after their birth, very calm and alert, very present and exceedingly peaceful beings.

Many of these young children believe they are here purely to teach others about love and to help us remember who we are on a spiritual level—that we are not just physical beings but spiritual beings as well.

In 2003 the remedy Pink Flannel Flower was made and I received the message that it was to be used for all children under the age of five, to keep open their heart chakras. These 'new millennium' children arrive with their hearts open but it is not always easy to keep them so when dealing with some of the harsher, crueller realities of our world. Yet it is vitally important that they are able to keep their hearts open, for it is much easier to be open spiritually and psychically when your heart chakra is expanded. A good percentage of these children are very sensitive and are very open emotionally; their feeling centres are quite well developed. They are moving away from the intellectual paradigm that has operated for the last few centuries. Many adults observing these young children look at them and think 'What very old souls'— and indeed they are.

We are now seeing what used to be known as the mystics and seers come back to bring gifts, talents and skills that have not been around for a very, very long time. These children are certainly far more evolved than previous generations, with many remembering who they were in past lives and where they were originally from. Many also remember Spirit and being back there in the spirit realm between their earthly lives.

Yet these children need the legacy of that earlier bridging generation, or 'indigo children' as some people call them. For these were the ones who came down to be warrior-like in preparing the most suitable environment for, as well as protecting, the younger children born since 2000. The children of the bridging generation won't obediently do as they are told if they can't see the point of it. If they see injustice they stand up against it. They challenge the accepted order, unlike any other generation before them. Their role has been a very important one: to prepare the way for the younger children coming through.

I am very optimistic about the future of our planet, for when these children with their inherent qualities of intuition, sensitivity and cooperation mature and reach positions of influence in government, education, business and the arts, they will be able to greatly influence our society in a very positive way. This will, hopefully, be in direct contrast to the twentieth century, which was the most violent, bloody century in the history of humanity with well over 100 million people killed violently in war and ethnic cleansing. The children coming through now are our hope and our future and I see the role of Bush Essences as one of assistance in helping these children fulfil their highest potential and destiny.

All the children born in this century will have at least one zero, which equates to spiritual potential, in their birth date. Many will have two or more zeros. Bush Essences, especially Meditation Essence, are wonderful tools to help activate this potential.

PERCEIVED LEARNING PROBLEMS

These children will face many challenges. The old academic teaching paradigms don't fit with them very well. Many are having, or will have, learning problems, though part of the reason so many children are labelled or diagnosed with ADHD is incomprehension on the part of 'experts' as to why traditional learning methods don't work for these children. These children are usually very bright and they get quickly bored with our old, outdated learning methods. They appear to have a short attention span because they can quickly grasp ideas and then move on to something else, and they often find retrieving information for exams is wearisome. They tend to compartmentalise a lot of information without displaying the same logical, intellectual, left-brain sequence most adults exhibit. These children also tend to operate more with telepathic communication. When young, they are sometimes labelled as having learning problems because they can be lazy in bothering to speak. Often they can startle adults when they do decide to speak and come out with full sentences. Cognis Essence should be the first treatment used for any child struggling in the classroom, whether it be with reading, spelling, maths or keeping up generally. The results with this remedy are exceptional—nothing that I have used or come across comes close to it.

Problems at school

Katie has always been a bright, happy girl. As a toddler she seemed to run everywhere—she was also slightly clumsy, falling over her feet every now and then. Katie has always had a good relationship with her parents and is very happy at home. When she started preschool she slotted in very well, then she started 'big school' and found kindergarten just like preschool.

In her second year of school Katie started misbehaving at school and at home—just little things at first like not listening in class or being cheeky to her parents. She also seemed to be rushing everywhere again—not stopping long enough to take anything in. Her mother learned from her teacher that Katie was struggling with her schoolwork, and also noticed that her reading at home had seemed to slump.

I gave Katie Cognis Essence. After three days Katie's mother was very excited about the change—she had slowed right down, was willing to help out around the house and had stopped being cheeky. Katie's teacher was amazed at the sudden change in Katie's behaviour and concentration. She was now eager to learn, and her reading had improved and was enjoyable again.

On a second consultation, we decided to give her a break from the Cognis Essence and have found that giving Katie the essence every two months for two weeks works well and that she is more than happy to take it as she knows it makes her 'learn better and be happier'.

Sue Nelson, New South Wales, Australia

SPIRITUAL ABILITIES

Another great challenge such children face is that in many cases parents won't be nearly as evolved spiritually as their children nor necessarily recognise their gifts or know the best ways to help their child develop them. The very powerful healing love vibrations these children bring through with them will also act as a catalyst to help develop the psychic awareness of others around them. However, if the children with these psychic abilities are not encouraged to use them or are ridiculed, or their parents don't understand what they are talking about, they can learn to switch them off. They may try to please their teachers or parents and conform to be like other children who don't have these gifts (and not all children are born with them). They will certainly look like other children but they will be very different from other children. And they too are, in a fashion, a bridging generation in helping to expand awareness so that what each future generation remembers, knows and does will be more and more commonplace.

Little Flannel Flower is a remedy to help restore those spiritual abilities in a child. However, if there is suppression then, according to Meg Losey in her book *The Children Of Now*, when these children grow older there is concern that they can develop self-worth issues, depression, feelings of insignificance, even sometimes what we would label autism, as they switch off from our reality into their own world.

The new millennium children are very spiritually gifted. Many are clairvoyant and have the ability to tune in to the more subtle realms that most adults don't even recognise or understand. So many of these children have a strong affinity with Nature, while others have a natural aptitude for computers and technology. As Jan Thomas writes, 'computers and nature have one thing in common, they are both worlds in worlds and each one is complete'.

Such children have great compassion and many are very good natural healers who often want to help others, though they can get quite tired, or even exhausted, as they take on the healing and the pain of those around them. These young children experience all their emotions very strongly and are very empathetic, feeling the hurt and suffering of others around them. They get very upset when other people are violent or are in emotional or physical pain.

These children will bring down new techniques and methods of healing. They will be less and less drawn to practices of healing and medicine that have many negative side effects as they are, by nature, very sensitive and adversely affected by such treatments.

There is a wise old adage which is especially appropriate for these children: the greater the talent, the greater need for self-discipline and self-control. Here again Bush Essences, in particular Hibbertia, can be of great help in assisting a child to develop these qualities within themselves.

These children, though very sensitive, are not fragile—they have a great inner strength and they will need it. There is likely to be much reluctance towards the new ideas and concepts they bring forth—people don't like change. Again, this is where the bridging generation who, now the oldest in their late twenties, will do a great job in preparing the soil for these new concepts and ideas. A lot of the young children will also have (and this is going to be quite crucial for the survival of this planet) not only a love and respect for Earth but also a willingness to fight to preserve Nature, our fauna, flora and our environment. These children will not want to fight Earth but help prepare it and work with it and understand it at a level we haven't seen for a long time. They will greatly enjoy doing rituals for healing and helping Earth, and have innate knowledge about how to help others and the planet.

Australian Bush Flower Essences are especially suited for this current generation of very loving, gentle, spiritually gifted children. They respond wonderfully to the higher vibration present in Bush Essences. These essences will help them adjust to a rapidly changing society, where their sensitivity and intuition will be more and more valued, appreciated and honoured.

A CHILD'S SPIRITUAL DEVELOPMENT

The following is a brief summary of some of the major spiritual developments of children.

Before a child incarnates they reside in the spirit world, resting between incarnations. It's a realm of rest for her soul and re-integration of her Higher Self. In the spirit world a soul learns from higher teachers and greater spirits, who give not only a great amount of perspective on their last life but even on other life cycles as well. It's here in the spirit world that the being will develop an outline or destiny pattern for their new incarnation.

When physical conception occurs the energy of that conception enters the spirit realm, where it is immediately noted, experienced and felt. Within that instant, everything about the two parents is perceived in the spirit world; the environment they live in, their genetic patterns, race, financial situation, belief systems, their thoughts, feelings, religion, even what's going on within the world and in the universe at that time. It's akin to a computer readout of every salient aspect pertaining to that conception. A spiritual being wishing to reincarnate will perceive that energy and if it has all the components it needs it will assign itself to that conception.

The pattern or blueprint has to be exactly right for the being wanting to come down; even if only one aspect of the energy pattern is unsuitable, that may be sufficient for the spirit not to choose that incarnation. For example, if parents live merely 10 kilometres away from an ideal location, this could mean the reincarnating spirit is unable to meet and have karmic relationships with hundreds of people. If it's a perfect match the spirit will send an energy force and seal the conception. Sometimes the soul, which is the person or that spirit made up of all her lifetimes, memories and personality, may not actually incarnate into the mother's body right at conception. The incarnation can occur anytime throughout the pregnancy although the being will be watching and observing. The soul is more likely to incarnate at the point of conception if it is a child's first lifetime or if it might have Down syndrome (which is usually its first incarnation where it is coming to observe and experience with very little responsibility).

As mentioned before, during her first three years a child's closest and most important relationship is with her mother. Health problems the child can have during this time may well reflect imbalances in the mother. From three to six years the bonding with, and influence of, the father takes on much greater importance. The child's illnesses may now also reflect imbalances in the father. It is not a bad idea when you give a remedy to a child to consider giving the same remedy to the mother or the father, depending on the child's age.

Between the ages of three to six is a very powerful time when a child can remember who and what she was in her previous life. She will identify with her past life now more than at any other time, though this influence will continue to be present until her ninth year. Often she will act out through her games and play what she was involved in during a past life. If such games or play are suppressed she may end up merely repeating the same pattern from her last lifetime and not developing fully. From six to nine there will be accentuation of the child's most recent lifetime and a scattering of interest in almost every lifetime they've had. So don't discourage any interest or hobby that they may pursue even briefly during this time. From nine to twelve there will be a lessening impact of that lifetime.

During the first twelve years a child displays great spiritual awareness, usually way beyond the understanding of her parents. It is a time when children will be able to commune and talk with their guardian angels and the Nature spirits. They will be aware of them, feel them and many will see them. By twelve these gifts are likely to leave, if the parents have not encouraged them or have been critical of them.

After twelve, the responsibility of the parents alters. By this point a child has pretty much learnt all she is going to learn from her parents, not only from what they have said but also what they have not said—by their actions, what they have done and not done. The best way parents can influence a child after age twelve is to love themselves. By the age of thirteen the child is what the parents have thought, felt and been, as well as what they have not thought, felt and been. At the age of thirteen children are very much on their own; they will make or break themselves from that point on, but who they are has been strongly influenced by those first twelve years. Beginning at thirteen they will start to branch out and experiment with what their parents have taught them.

Between the ages of thirteen and eighteen, the parents will see their own traits and imbalances mirrored within their child, which is often why many parents have difficulty with their teenagers. From nine to twelve you begin to see a liberation of the child taking steps away, but from thirteen to eighteen you see what the parents have created.

One of the great things with children is that the remedies work extremely quickly on them; they are very open to the essences, and they don't have as many blocks and barriers on the emotional and subconscious levels as adults do. Also, today's children are particularly fine-tuned and I find that the essences can work on them quicker than previous generations of children. Children also have an innate intuition: they are an old soul in a new mind and a new body.

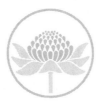

8

COMMON CHILDHOOD INFECTIONS AND ILLNESSES

After the first six months of life, the natural immunity your child has gained from breast milk tends to wear off. From that point onwards, especially up to the age of four, it's not uncommon for children to have a wide range of illnesses, many of which have fevers*. The majority of these illnesses are viral.

If your child is well looked after and very simple practices are put into place she will gain natural immunity from many illnesses. Apart from giving lots of love, one of the most important things you can do is to give your child reassurance and provide her with a sense of security. You can do this by showing confidence in your ability to look after her without rushing to a practitioner at the first sign of any symptom. She will then feel calm and, on a subconscious level, feel secure that you are able to help and heal her. This is where Australian Bush Flower Essences are very bencficial, as there are essences for just about every situation.

When your child is sick, don't send her to bed and isolate her. Keep her in contact with you. You'll find she gets better a lot quicker when she feels that safety, security and your love.

When you are treating a child with a fever, only give liquids, never milk but water or diluted fruit juice or very diluted lemonade. This will prevent any dehydration especially if there is also vomiting or diarrhoea. Fresh juices are always better than prepared juices. They have a lot more life force along with their nutrients and vitamins, and so are far more beneficial. She Oak is the remedy for dehydration: give 7 drops in each glass of liquid, which will help her absorb the liquid and stop dehydration.

Most children don't want to eat when they are sick. There is a misconception that parents need to keep their children's strength up by giving them more solid food or heavier liquids such as an egg flip. But it does no harm to a child not to eat solid food for a few days. When there is no food to digest, the body can use its blood to direct healing energies to where the problem is rather than having to expend energy digesting food. Once your child starts feeling better, provide a very light diet such as fruit.

If your child feels flat after an illness, Dynamis Essence will renew enthusiasm and pick her up. One of the remedies in this essence is Banksia Robur, which is for those who don't feel like their usual self and helps them recover from illnesses such as influenza*. That old energy and vitality will quickly come back. Another remedy in the essence is Illawarra Flame Tree, which will work on the thymus gland to help boost immunity.

ANTIBIOTICS

Antibiotics can have a serious effect on your child's wellbeing. Almost all of the infections from which children suffer are viral and will run their course. In the case of ear infections, consider avoiding antibiotics for the first two days, in which time most infections settle down. Extensive use of antibiotics in childhood can lead to an increase in asthma*. If your child has had antibiotics, follow up with Purifying Essence to release any toxins from the body.

Fortunately, these days doctors are less inclined to give antibiotics for conditions such as influenza* or sore throat*—they realise that they are viral and will not respond to antibiotics.

Being breastfed gives your child a good start, promoting healthy bacteria in the gut which keeps pathogens, other 'bad bacteria', yeasts, moulds and parasites in check. Antibiotics can wipe out colonies of good bacteria, as can a high-sugar diet. Green Essence can reharmonise that balance. To promote the growth of good bacteria, give your child the probiotics acidophilus and bifidus, which are available in powder form from health food stores. Buy only refrigerated probiotics and store them in your fridge. Give the probiotics with a little yoghurt to increase the colonies of good bacteria.

ASTHMA

Asthma* is a common chest problem for one in four Australian children, and it's a similar figure in other developed countries. Grief or sadness can often be the trigger for this illness, and it is sometimes associated with what is known as 'smother-love'. This is often seen in families where the mother's emotional needs are not met by the father and she tries to get them met from her children. Especially when this happens with a son there's a real sense of smothering, which can lead to asthma.

From the purely physical point of view, if I'm treating a child with asthma I always check their case history to see whether in the first year to eighteen months they had eczema which was treated with cortisone. The body in its wisdom tries to throw off metabolic waste through the skin. If the skin's elimination process is suppressed with cortisone creams you often find, two to three years later, asthma developing as a result. Purifying Essence is a very powerful skin cleanser, a very powerful detoxifier of the body, and it will help remove the effects of cortisone creams. It will need to be taken for at least one month.

Emergency Essence will help to release the muscle spasm and bronchiole constriction the occurs with asthma, and it will ease some of the terror if your child can't breathe. It will also help if the asthma is brought on by an environmental trigger, whether it's food, pollens, dust mites or chemical pollution. Emergency Essence decreases any sensitivity to that trigger.

In acute episodes give Emergency Essence to which Tall Mulla Mulla can be added, as often as every ten to fifteen minutes if the attack is very distressing. Tall Mulla Mulla essence is specific for breathing problems. Ongoing treatment would be with Tall Mulla Mulla.

Asthma

A young boy was suffering from asthma and his parents were unhappy about the drugs he had been prescribed. They didn't want him to use too many steroids because they knew that in the long term it could weaken the lungs. The boy was put on Purifying Essence to help remove the chemicals of the medication from his body and to help his lymphatic system, clearing out excessive mucus and toxins from the sinuses, throat and lungs. His acute attacks were successfully treated with

Emergency Essence. Tall Mulla Mulla and Fringed Violet were used as ongoing treatments and he rarely suffered from asthma.
Ian

If your baby was premature

Because the lungs are among the last organs to develop, a baby who is born prematurely may suffer from asthma or bronchial problems. The flower Tall Mulla Mulla is a very specific remedy for helping circulation of both breath and blood, and it is useful in these cases.

Asthma

I treated a young girl who had been sexually and mentally abused two years ago. She was fearful and suffered severe asthma and food allergies, was paranoid about spiders and had nightmares. I made up Grey Spider Flower to be given at the onset of an asthma attack, and hourly (or more often) until comfortable. Usually when she has an episode of asthma she needs a nebuliser every four hours for about a week. After the Grey Spider Flower the nebuliser was only used for a day and the severity of the attacks was reduced dramatically.

Rosemary Evans, New South Wales, Australia

AUTISM

In many Western countries, the current rate of Autism Spectrum Disorders (ASD) is about 1 in every 150 children, a much higher incidence than it was in previous generations. There is no cure nor still a clearly accepted reason why it occurs, however many believe there is a link with vaccinations, as was discussed in Chapter 5.

Some children today are classified as autistic when in fact they are just very different to others in their communication styles. However, there are still many children who display the common features of autism*. Usually they will exhibit very repetitive, obsessive behaviours, can be extremely attached to routines, get very upset and disturbed when things change, and react with a lot of rigidity to life's experiences. Many have difficulty with social interactions, communication and behaviour which are major, regular parts of life. Many autistic children have sensory sensitivities which can cause them to feel frustrated, fearful, anxious or confused.

Bush Fuchsia, found in both Calm and Clear Essence and Cognis Essence, is one of the most important remedies, as it gives one a sense of orientation. It will help these children relate to the outside world. Many children with autism have difficulty with speech, and many speech pathologists work with Bush Fuchsia to help them in communicating and speaking. Flannel Flower helps in expressing feelings and in making eye contact, Bauhinia helps facilitate acceptance and openness to change, while Emergency Essence is very good for fear and confusion. Wild Potato Bush helps with frustration and the inability to communicate or express themselves effectively, which often leads to physical aggression.

Diagnosis of ASD is not usually made until about two or three years of age. Early diagnosis and the appropriate forms of treatment, such as speech pathology, occupational therapy and behaviour intervention, are best started as early as possible. It is difficult to cure the condition of autism, however, as Elizabeth Curran, a parent who regularly works with Bush Essences for her two autistic boys, says: 'Consistency over time is my motto for working with autism. Sometimes it can take quite a long time to break through a behaviour and release a pattern, a ritual or obsession.' In working with Bush Flower Essences, Elizabeth has found there have been effective shifts in her sons.

In writing about children, Doreen Virtue says that many young children today, whom she calls 'crystal children', are being diagnosed as autistic partly because they go into trances and are oblivious to what's going on around them. In her research she has noticed that this seems to happen when the children are outdoors, in Nature. A similar pattern occurs in autistic children, although she makes the distinction that the children she calls crystal children are incredibly affectionate, with a great deal of empathy, and they are connected with other people. Although from time to time they do tune out the outside world, but it is only temporary. Sundew can help bring someone back to earth and ground such episodes.

In her book *Children Now*, Meg Losey discusses her belief that many physically gifted children who are not recognised or encouraged in their abilities withdraw into their own alternate realities about which they have difficulty communicating in everyday language. She believes that the discomfort with touch experienced by so-called autistic children is due to their extreme sensitivity—they are like physic sponges and absorb all the feelings and experiences that the person touching them has ever had. For such sensitive children Fringed Violet is imperative and will afford them greater psychic protection. Losey also feels that in autistic children the pathways of electromagnetic energy within their brains become caught in a loop. The energy moves in a circular or elliptical pattern in a small area of their brains, while the sensory receptors get stuck on 'go'. This can cause the network of neurons within the brain to develop a small, restricted format. This can lead to the varying degrees of autism and it is, Losey believes, why some of the most severely affected, the 'savants', are able to be geniuses in a specific area. Bush Fuchsia would be the most appropriate essence for this.

Autism

My son, Marcus, has been an extremely stubborn child with his autism. He refused to learn to ride a bike, becoming frustrated because he could not do it right away. The result was tantrums, big time. I put him on Isopogon and this has helped to break down his rigidity to learn the skill of bike riding. Bike riding has been a great skill for him to learn, making him very independent. Isopogon has helped a lot in chipping away the extremes of his behaviour. He is more flexible now rather than just rigid.

Elizabeth Curran, Victoria, Australia

Refusal to change

I have also worked with Freshwater Mangrove for over a year on and off with Marcus. It seems to be the perfect essence for him in many ways. Marcus is unaware of his 'no good reason' for not trying new things. Marcus has a lot of rigidities in his responses to life experiences and it is very challenging for him to let go and choose to do things differently. He has a rigid preference for certain colours and clothes as well as food. I believe it is his fear of the future which makes him need a lot of familiarity. This essence has helped him let go of some of his refusal to change and helped him break this pattern and introduce a few new colours to his apparel. Marcus is fascinated with black hair. Two students in his class have shiny black hair. Marcus wears sunglasses a lot, so as not to make eye contact and yet in front of the whole class he allowed the class to help him dye his hair black. He does not usually like to be visible and in this case he was the centre of attention. I thought this example of the effect of the essence was amazing, such a rigid boy in many ways and the experience of the hair dyeing was an unexpected breakthrough. The perceptual shifts from this essence are helping him to identify the world outside of himself.

Elizabeth Curran, Victoria, Australia

Autism

After a workshop with Ian, I gave my son, a non-verbal autistic, Bush Fuchsia. Immediately, the school he attends told me he was having good days. Within two weeks they asked me what I had done and to keep doing it. Within a few weeks he started to point at things and to respond to instruction. He started cycling forward on a bike that he now loves. He was vocalising much more, playing with age-appropriate toys and starting to join in with other children which all the other mums commented on. The list is becoming endless, almost every day he does something new.

Ruth Goodman, United Kingdom

Dyspraxia

My great niece is three and has not made any sound. She has been diagnosed as dyspraxic. She cannot copy sounds although her understanding and ability to follow instructions is well advanced. She was getting quite downhearted, not willing to try as it was too hard. I followed Ian's suggestion and after a month of taking Cognis Essence she now has 100 words, still indistinct but nevertheless progress is being made steadily. What her mum says is that the most important thing she has noticed since taking Cognis is that she is now willing to try and say any word whereas before she was not.

Jan Brumfritt, United Kingdom

Autism

One of my clients has four sons, three diagnosed with autism. She decided to try flower essences for her most severely affected child, her six year old. I gave her a bottle of Cognis Essence with the addition of Flannel Flower and Yellow Cowslip Orchid to be taken morning and night. Before taking the essences the little boy had a vocabulary of eight words, was not fully toilet trained, and screamed when asked to do something he didn't want to do.

One week later a very excited mother came to see me. Her child's vocabulary had increased to thirty words including the names of family members, the teacher and some kids at kindy. When asked to do something he didn't want to do, he responded firmly but calmly, 'No, no, no.' He had become more interested in people, making better eye contact and repeating words and phrases. He started toileting independently. A second bottle led to him settling in well to his new school and steady progress in all areas of learning and development including a marked escalation in his writing and its legibility.

Margaret Yarnton, Victoria, Australia

BRONCHITIS

Bronchitis* affects the lungs, which in Chinese medicine are associated with grief and sadness. Bronchial or asthmatic problems can develop after the death or loss of someone close, or even a loved pet. Sturt Desert Pea specifically addresses such grief.

Once you deal with the grief, the physical body starts to heal itself. Give your child a light diet and avoid any dairy foods, which is essential in any condition where there is excess mucus such as hay fever, sinus problems, colds etc.

A good indication of how your child's lungs are improving is whether he sleeps through the 3 a.m. to 5 a.m. period. In Chinese medicine this is 'lung time', so if there is a problem with the lungs the symptoms often get worse during this time and the child will wake.

CHICKEN POX

This is a viral condition that starts with a mild fever* and is followed by a rash that spreads, the lesions filling with fluid and forming small blisters. After a few days these burst and scab over, which can cause scarring if scratched. It can be difficult stopping children from scratching because the rash is itchy.

Chicken pox

My daughter developed a high temperature with delirium at night, and the next day had a red rash over her torso and behind her neck. The spots were very itchy. After the delirium attack I gave her Emergency Essence and kept it up every hour for three hours. After the first dose the delirium subsided within minutes and the fever dropped dramatically in the next hour. The essence addressed the panic, fear and distress in my child. The next day I gave her one dose of the essences listed for chicken pox and I gave her Spinifex, applying it directly to her itchy rash. The itching stopped straight away. The next morning there were no signs of spots.

Amanda Saunders, Victoria, Australia

Spinifex is a remedy specific for blistering lesions. Chicken pox* is connected to the herpes virus, and Spinifex works on cold sores on the mouth and genitals, as well as shingles. A bad case of chicken pox can predispose a child to these conditions later in life. Spinifex, applied both internally and topically, will usually stop or dramatically reduce the itch. Billy Goat Plum helps with any sense of revulsion about the scabs and how the child feels when looking at their rash. Both Emergency Essence and Wild Potato Bush can help a child deal with any frustration and irritation they may feel when they have chicken pox.

Skin rashes

In my 'Mother's Survival Kit' would be Spinifex which is invaluable in assisting all forms of skin rash. From nappy rash to chick pox it is amazing in healing, reducing inflammation and itching and preventing scarring. In fact I make sure that my children have Spinifex in their bath on a regular basis and I believe it speeds the healing of old scratches, scrapes and blisters (all of which are a daily occurrence with boisterous boys of this age, three and five). I've given it to other young mothers who verify the amazing impact on nappy rash and chicken pox in particular.

Janne Ferguson, Victoria, Australia

Fungal infections

My seven-year-old daughter was suffering from a very nasty fungal infection on both her feet, between the toes the skin was wounded, open and very bad smelling. She also had a deep wart under the right heel. I gave her a foot bath in tepid water with drops of Green Essence every morning for five minutes. After three weeks of treatment the fungal infection was healed, the wart took longer but now it is completely gone. During the time of treatment she had very strange, strong nightmares, it was like the Green Essence worked very deeply removing every kind of disturbance, physical ones and emotional too! Thanks a lot.

Lorenzo Avanzato, Belgium

Warts

My daughter had a lot of warts on her hands and was being teased at school about them. Just when I thought I'd exhausted all possibilities for getting rid of them, I remembered Green Essence. My daughter applied it topically. It was a slow process and took a few months to be rid of them completely, but it was wonderful watching them shrink into nothing. My daughter was so happy to be able to show her hands again without being teased.

Dawn Detmers, Queensland, Australia

COLDS

The common symptoms of a cold are a sore throat*, slight tenderness in the ear and coughs*. These can cause a lot of discomfort, and Emergency Essence will ease the pain. For sore ears you can rub some Bush Fuchsia around the mastoid bone, the bone just behind the ear. Bush Fuchsia is shaped like a trumpet and is good for all ear complaints.

Give your child plenty of fluids along with lots of love and reassurance. The remedies listed in Chapter 14 for influenza apply to colds, too. Basically, they help a child to recover from being run-down or overwhelmed, boosting her immune system and stimulating the lymphatics, the body's defence mechanism.

EARACHE

For quick relief of pain or discomfort associated with earache, apply some drops of Emergency Essence internally and also topically to the mastoid bone, which is just behind the ear.

Some children who have chronic ear infections develop otitis media, commonly known as 'glue ear'. Sticky fluid builds up in the middle ear and over time can affect a child's hearing and consequently their learning. Grommets have often been inserted to treat glue ear, but medical studies now indicate these are not effective. However, Bush Fuchsia is very effective for chronic ear infections.

If your child suffers a lot of ear problems, be aware of whether there is a lot of arguing going on at home. Maybe there is an older, teenage child arguing with you or your partner, or maybe it's the parents themselves arguing with each other. A new child can represent a lot of stress in a family and sometimes that stress can manifest in more fighting than normal, especially if the parents are tired and not getting enough sleep.

Ear infections

Mandy (not her real name) presented to me as a pale, frail, listless seven-year-old prone to frequent bad ear infections. She was often visiting a doctor and taking prescriptions for antibiotics. She had missed a lot of school, having not spent one full week in education for almost a year. I prescribed Red Grevillea for infection and her sense of 'stuckness', Bush Fuchsia for the head and especially the ears and Bottlebrush for the pain and also to help the communication with her mother. She was the youngest of two children and recently her brother had been receiving a great deal of attention, so Illawarra Flame Tree was given to support her immune system and help with any feelings of rejection. After three days the pain was diminishing but the ear was still discharging and she was able to sleep at night. Two days later she said she felt a lot better and had a little sparkle in her eye and was wanting to play with others. In another three days the ear had stopped running and her voice could be heard in all corners of the house, a sure sign the child was recovering. Two weeks later Mandy had spent her first whole week at school in a very long time, continuing with her drops there have been no ear infections for many months, her sleeping is sounder, she has more vitality and she has taken up gymnastic classes.

Practitioner's name supplied but withheld on request

GERMAN MEASLES

German measles* produces a very fine rash, and can be accompanied by fever* and a general unwell feeling. Give Mulla Mulla for the fever and Emergency Essence for feeling not quite right.

MEASLES

Measles* can be a debilitating condition. It usually begins with a runny nose, coughs*, a sore throat* and fever*, and is sometimes mistaken for a cold or bronchitis. A child can be quite sick with measles, vomiting and suffering abdominal pain. Your child becomes infectious about three days after the rash appears. The remedy Mulla Mulla will keep the fever in check, and Emergency Essence will help ease any pain and distress.

MUMPS

Mumps* is a viral condition that results in swelling of the parotid salivary glands, which lie at the back of the cheek between the ear and the jaw. The condition can be painful, but it is not usually a very severe illness. The Bush Essence Hibbertia is specific for the parotid salivary glands and will help ease the swelling there.

One complication of mumps in boys can be inflammation of the testes, although this is not very common. If a boy gets mumps, give him Flannel Flower for protection of the testes.

WORMS

Worms are a common condition in children. A clue that your child has worms is that she has dark circles under her eyes, feels tired and complains of an itchy bottom. Sometimes you can even see the worms, usually pin worms, coming out in the child's stools. The symptoms seem to be worse at night, when your child unconsciously scratches her anus.

Green Essence taken internally is very good for helping to eliminate any parasites in the body. Purifying Essence can also be used. Because sugar creates a good breeding ground for parasites in the intestines, it is a good idea to decrease the amount of sugar in your child's diet. The remedy Bottlebrush is a very effective detoxifier for the large intestine. Increasing the healthy bacteria is also a good idea, so give acidophilus and bifidus. These are available in the refrigerator section of health food shops. Make sure to keep them refrigerated at home.

Alpine Mint Bush

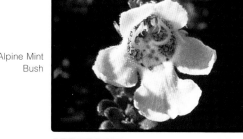

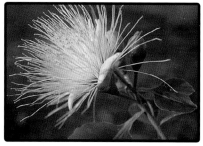

Billy Goat Plum

Angelsword

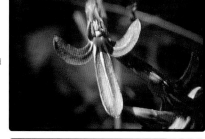

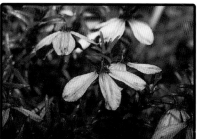

Black-eyed Susan

Autumn Leaves

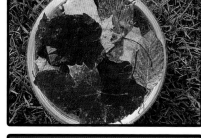

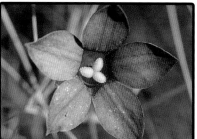

Bluebell

Banksia Robur

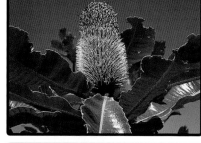

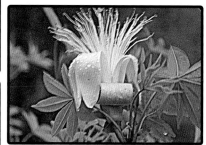

Boab

Bauhinia

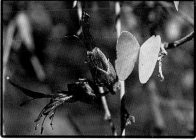

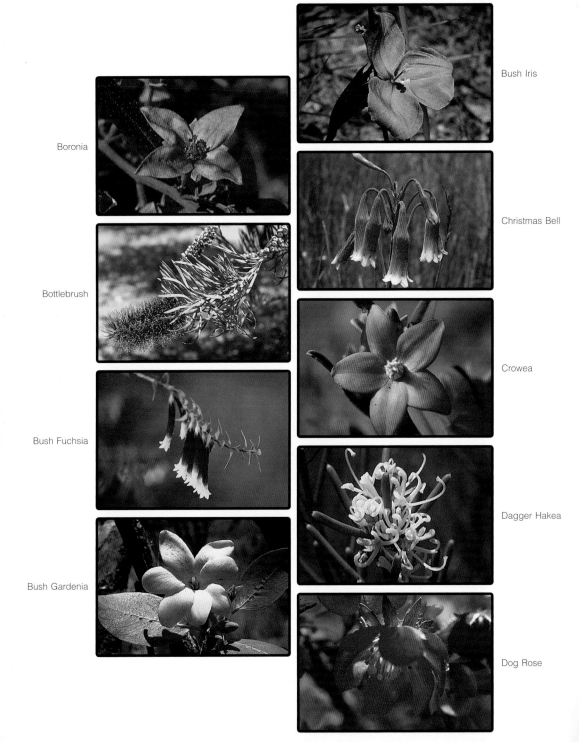

Boronia

Bottlebrush

Bush Fuchsia

Bush Gardenia

Bush Iris

Christmas Bell

Crowea

Dagger Hakea

Dog Rose

Dog Rose of the Wild Forces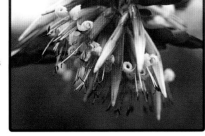

Green Essence

Five Corners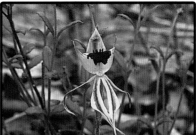

Green Spider Orchid

Flannel Flower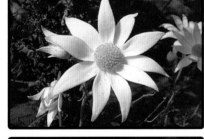

Grey Spider Flower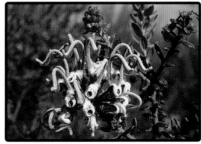

Freshwater Mangrove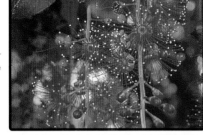

Gymea Lily

Fringed Violet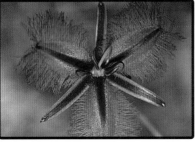

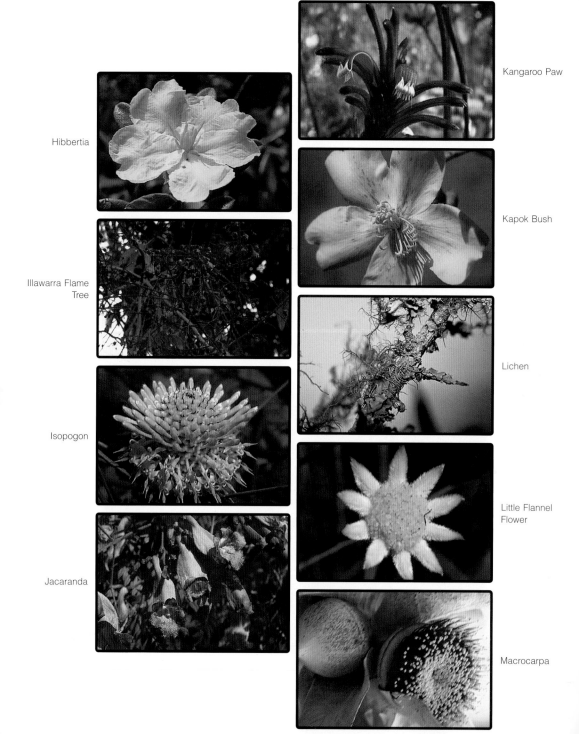

Hibbertia

Illawarra Flame Tree

Isopogon

Jacaranda

Kangaroo Paw

Kapok Bush

Lichen

Little Flannel Flower

Macrocarpa

Mint Bush

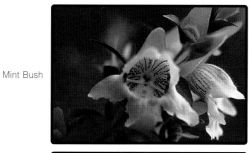

Monga Waratah

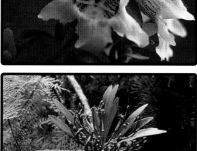

Mountain Devil

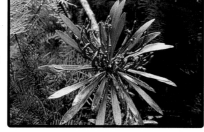

Mulla Mulla

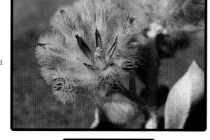

Old Man
Banksia

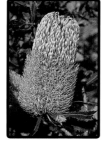

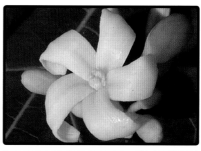

Paw Paw

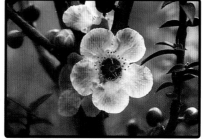

Peach-flowered
Tea-tree

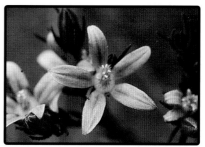

Philotheca

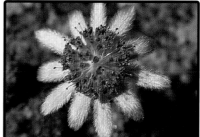

Pink Flannel
Flower

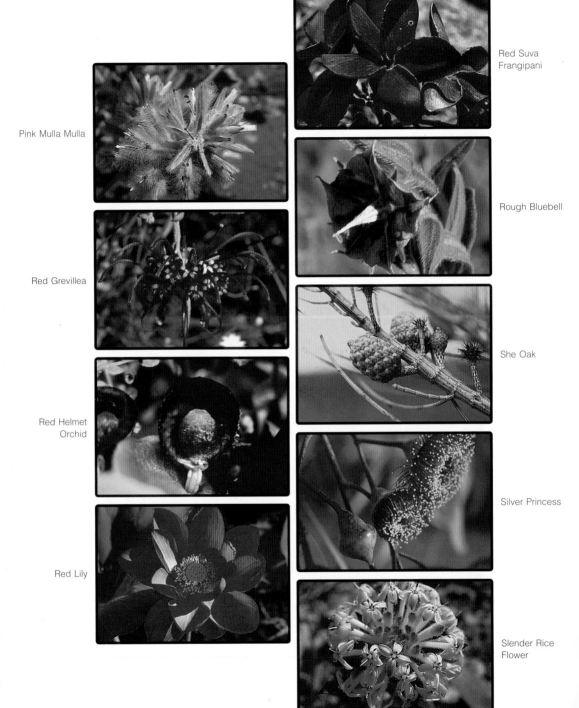

Pink Mulla Mulla

Red Suva
Frangipani

Red Grevillea

Rough Bluebell

Red Helmet
Orchid

She Oak

Silver Princess

Red Lily

Slender Rice
Flower

Southern Cross

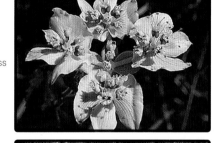

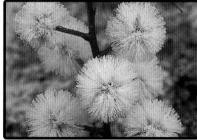

Sunshine Wattle

Spinifex

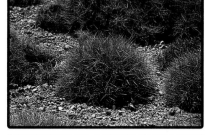

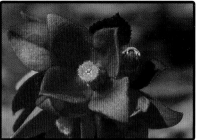

Sydney Rose

Sturt Desert Pea

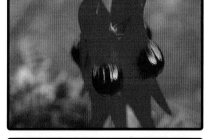

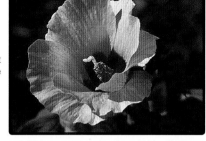

Tall Mulla Mulla

Sturt Desert Rose

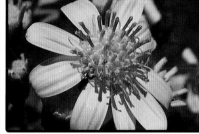

Tall Yellow Top

Sundew

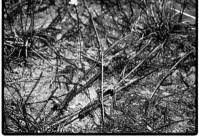

Turkey Bush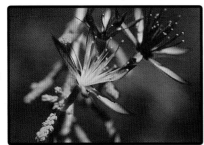

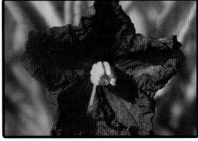 Wild Potato
Bush

Waratah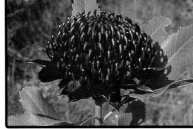

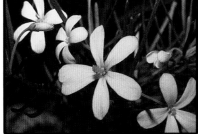 Wisteria

Wedding Bush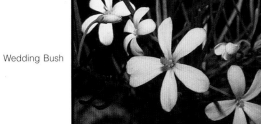

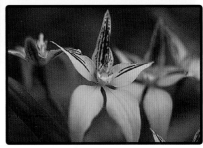 Yellow Cowslip
Orchid

If you have pets, your child may be in close physical contact with them, even kissing them. You only have to see your dog chewing its own faeces, sniffing the bottom of another dog or licking itself clean to realise how easily parasites can be passed on. For this reason, to keep parasites at bay give your child a dose of Green Essence for two weeks every six months or so.

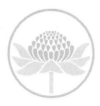

9

TODDLERHOOD TO CHILDHOOD

During this stage, between three and five years of age, your child will become more and more independent. Gradually she will start to play with other children, and once she starts daycare or preschool you'll notice how other people in her life start to influence her. All the same, her mum and dad remain the most important people in her life. Allow her the opportunity to explore and learn more about her world, and try to step back a little. She continues to need your unconditional love and your protection, but she also needs to try things for herself. This is the way a baby moves into early childhood. The more she feels she can do for herself the more confident she will feel, as long as she knows that you are always there.

PLAYING IN THE NATURAL WORLD

All kinds of play arc absolutely essential for a child's development, and one of the best places for children to play is in the natural environment. When they are young, children relate to the world through their senses and through moving their bodies, and being outside in the open air allows for all this. This generation of children will both crave and benefit from being in Nature more than previous generations.

Many children these days do a lot of sitting, either in front of a computer screen or in front of a television. What they need for good health is plenty of play outdoors. In fact, some of the most influential people in the field of early childhood development, such as Steiner and Montessori, believed that children need to have direct interaction with the natural world through playing there. The home environment today is too stimulating for many children and it affects the development of their brains. Playing in Nature helps to restore some balance.

Grounding

From the time he began to walk, Travis would get around on tiptoes. He was given Cognis Essence, because it contains Bush Fuchsia, to address his coordination, and Sundew, to help ground him.
Ian

Playing in the natural world doesn't have to be dangerous. It can mean digging up weeds, examining the work of ants, running and skipping in the local park, following the buzz of insects. If your child sees you enjoying Nature and its bounty, she'll learn to appreciate it in the same way.

For parents: Being playful

The remedy Little Flannel Flower will help you get in touch with your own playfulness, giving you a sense of being carefree and joyous. It's a wonderful remedy if you find it difficult to join your child in the fun of play.
Ian

MAKING FRIENDS

At this stage children tend to keep to other children they know, either through preschool or daycare, or because they are the children of your friends or neighbours. If you ask a child of this age who her friends are, she'll tell you the names of children she plays with the most. Your child is in the process of learning the 'rules' of relationships, and she will watch you more than you realise. If your child tends to keep to herself, don't worry about it or try to force friendships onto her. Some children are less sociable than others at this age, and they need time to establish friendships with others.

FORMING BASIC BELIEFS

By the time we are three years old, most of our basic beliefs about life have already been formed and stored in our subconscious. Even while still in the womb we are absorbing experiences and establishing an orientation to life, and these beliefs continue to guide and direct our actions throughout adulthood.

For example, a very young child might have overly concerned parents who constantly hover over her and step in to do everything for her 'in case she gets hurt'. As she grows older she may have no conscious memory of this early experience but the message that life is dangerous and she is under constant threat may have been stored as a belief, which will influence her frequently during the rest of her life during which she will unconsciously create situations that reinforce this belief. For example, every time a new opportunity is presented to her she may shrink back in fear and become increasingly timid about trying new things. She may also expect other people to step in to help her.

The frustrating part about this situation is that the person doesn't consciously know why she shrinks back, and doesn't realise that her fear is caused by her belief that she is unable to protect herself from possible hurt.

Of course, positive beliefs are also stored in the subconscious mind. They may be beliefs like 'I am a caring human being', or 'People love me even if I get angry', or 'Life is fun'. Parents have a wonderful opportunity—and responsibility—to help develop positive beliefs in their children. Confid Essence is a fantastic essence to assist parents in this goal. Containing the remedy Five Corners, this combination is able to clear negative beliefs from the subconscious.

FAMILY PATTERNS

You may begin to notice, when your child is around this age, that family patterns start to emerge in them. You may notice that things you or someone else in the family does are coming through in your child. For example, when my daughter was very small, we were driving somewhere together and I was going a little fast, speeding up, feeling impatient because we were running late. She was chatting away, and I noticed that she was become zingy: she was talking faster and getting worked up. I can remember thinking: 'Oh no, she'll grow up like me', and as soon as we got home I started her on a course of Boab, *the* remedy to clear family patterns. Children basically learn and play out behavioural patterns and idiosyncrasies—good and not so good—of their parents from the earliest age.

SIBLING RIVALRY

Between the ages of three and five, many children have a new sibling or two arrive on the scene. Some children take it in their stride, but most have some form of reaction. There are many possible remedies for sibling rivalry*, depending on the particular situation. The main remedy is Mountain Devil for jealousy.

Another good remedy for sibling rivalry is Bluebell, which opens the heart and helps a child share all resources, including toys and parents. If your child tries to get a sibling into trouble, such as crying when he is not really hurt and blaming his brother, then Rough Bluebell is the remedy for such manipulation. It is also the appropriate remedy for extreme violence and cruelty. I have successfully treated young children with this remedy who have attempted to smother or even drown their new sibling!

Aggressive behaviour

Mark was an energetic three-and-a-half-year-old who was becoming nasty towards everyone, especially his new baby sister. Some of the Bush Flowers I prescribed were:

- Illawarra Flame Tree to ease feelings of rejection, as his mum was now spending a lot of time with the new baby;
- Flannel Flower for gentleness towards his new sister;

- Mountain Devil to clear away anger and let his inherent love come through; and
- Rough Bluebell to stop him being hurtful to his sister and mother.

After three days, Mark's mother said she had back the son she knew and loved.

Jill Ramsden, United Kingdom

Unsettled behaviour

Carlin was a cheerful, playful child until the birth of his sister. He became clingy and cried about everything. He also started fighting at school and teachers and the parents of other children started complaining. I recommended:

- Mountain Devil for the jealousy and the aggression he felt; and
- Kangaroo Paw to be more sensitive and less self-focused.

Within days Carlin was cheerful again and he had changed so much that he wanted to do everything for his sister and helped his mother bathe his sister. His mother said he was back to the normal little boy she knew.

Esmerelda Robinson, United Arab Emirates

YOUR CHILD'S SAFETY

Sometimes what your child wants to do can be a threat to his safety. He doesn't want to be under supervision, for example, but wants to run across the street on his own. For the sake of your child's safety you have to take charge, so there can be battles of will with your child defying your authority. This is especially the case as your child approaches three and four years old. At this age children need to realise that they can't get everything they want, and they have to be considerate of other people and their needs. If your child is overly focused on his own needs at three or four years of age, then Kangaroo Paw will help him. It engenders kindness, awareness and sensitivity towards other people. Red Helmet Orchid will help with authority issues.

'Unsociable' behaviour

Michelle was a three-and-a-half-year-old whose behaviour was 'unsociable', according to her mother. She was bright and active, and always prepared to be in charge. I suggested she select some cards, and she chose:

- Bottlebrush to improve the mother–child bond;
- Black-eyed Susan to slow down and have patience; and
- Rough Bluebell to transform spite and manipulation into love and compassion.

Soon after treatment began, Michelle was more relaxed and her mother reported her tantrums had become much shorter. She also felt more connected with her daughter.

Cheryl Hingerty, New South Wales, Australia

DEMANDING BEHAVIOUR

For a number of different reasons children can become very demanding*, relentlessly seeking attention from one or both of their parents. Two of the basic needs of children are unconditional love along with plenty of attention, and if these needs are not met adequately they can become sick to get attention. Give the remedy Gymea Lily if your child always wants to be the centre of attention, speaking over other people and trying to dominate the situation. If you sense that your child is demanding because he feels insecure, give Dog Rose.

A demanding child

Sometimes your child will be demanding because she knows that eventually you will give in. If this is the case you would benefit from Flannel Flower, which will help you to establish healthy boundaries.

Ian

DISINTEREST IN FOOD

Children can become disinterested in food for a number of reasons. Sometimes they are a little bit vague and spacey; childhood education pioneer Rudolph Steiner believed children are not fully incarnated in their bodies until the age of seven. Sundew is a remedy to help ground your child and bring her back into her body, into the physical, which may make her more interested in food.

When your child shows a disinterest in food and eating, make sure there are not too many distractions going on. Remedies in Calm and Clear Essence can help here: if your child is easily distracted, Jacaranda will help her focus more on eating, and Black-eyed Susan will calm her down so that she is more in the mood to eat.

If any foods are causing bad reactions children may become disinterested in eating, so treat for allergies* or food intolerance*. Dark circles under the eyes are an indication of such problems.

Calm mealtimes

Get into the habit of turning off the television during mealtimes so that the family can focus on eating. Some families eat dinner while watching the news at night, but some of the images can be very upsetting for children, and this can cause digestive problems.

Ian

Mealtime stress

A three-year-old girl suffered a vomiting attack during a meal, and even months later, whenever there was the slightest stress during a meal, she would gag on her food and vomit. Otherwise she was a healthy child. She was given Emergency Essence morning and night and when necessary at mealtimes. Within two weeks the problem was resolved. After four months,

there had been no recurrence and her mother noted that the little girl was more confident and less clingy than before she'd taken the essence.
Wanda Amos, New South Wales, Australia

WHINGEING

A whingeing tone of voice is usually learnt. It can indicate that your child is feeling like a victim, complaining that things are unfair. She feels helpless because she is unable to get what she wants. The essence Southern Cross is the remedy for when she feels a sense of being a victim.

Of course one of the big problems is that whingeing children can grow up into whingeing adults. If your child tends to whinge, when he is a bit older you can ask him to talk clearly in his normal tone of voice for what he wants.

Whingeing
Parents have told me that after using Rough Bluebell their children stopped whingeing and whining. It helps to curb their desire to manipulate and use their tone of voice in an attempt to get what they want.
Ian

TIME IN THE SUN

You may be very concerned about your child being exposed to sunlight, but children do need some sun for vitamin D production. If your child doesn't get enough vitamin D, she can have problems with her auto-immune system. If you're worried about sunburn or sun damage give her a dose of Solaris Essence before going outdoors. Not getting enough exposure to sunlight can also affect the pineal gland, which is normally activated by light. The remedy Bush Iris, which is in Purifying Essence, can help with this. This is especially the case in winter, when your child may not be getting a lot of sunlight because there's been a lot of rain and she has been indoors, or if she has been sick. Bush Iris will help activate the pineal gland in all situations.

Improving sunblock

One albino family in Argentina reported that they were badly burnt every summer no matter how much sunblock they used. They started to work with Mulla Mulla orally and putting it on along with the sunblock, and found they no longer got burnt.

Ian

TRAVELLING

Bush Iris is one of the main components of the combination Travel Essence. I recommend this combination be taken hourly while flying as it will negate many of the negative effects you are exposed to when travelling by plane. Bush Iris works on the pineal gland and will help regulate your body clock and assist in adjusting to different time zones, thereby greatly minimising any impact of jet lag. Travel Essence can also be taken by children who get motion sickness from boats or cars. The remedies Paw Paw and Crowea in the essence prevent and take away nausea. Emergency Essence is also fantastic for anyone with a fear of flying. It works brilliantly. Take some Emergency Essence in the days leading up to a flight and give to your child as often as needed while flying.

Easy travelling

Recently on my trip to Bali I used Travel Essence for the first time and loved it, I didn't get travel sick at all in the car or plane, whereas when I went to Hong Kong I used ginger tablets and didn't travel too well. I have used the essences a lot over the years for myself, family, friends and clients and still get moments of amazement.

On the flight home there was a baby, approximately four months old, who was very distressed and crying before we took off. I offered the mother my Travel Essence to put on the baby's hands—well, the baby went off to sleep before we started taxiing for takeoff and slept all the way to Sydney and I did too. The mother couldn't believe it and thanked me when I got off at Sydney. The lady sitting next to me had to know what it was also so it was shared around. The rest of the passengers were suitably impressed.

Heidi Silver, Queensland, Australia

SURGERY

If a child is to have surgery, I always recommend they are given Emergency Essence for three days before the surgery and for a good two weeks afterwards. This essence will ease any fear and anxiety a child has about being separated from the family and having an operation. It will also ease the pain during recovery. To help the adrenal glands, which are badly affected by anaesthetics, you can add the remedy Macrocarpa.

Slender Rice Flower can also be added to Emergency Essence to help with the healing of scars. Held in the scar is any emotion you were feeling at the time of the surgery, or at the time of the accident if this is what caused the scarring. The great thing about Slender Rice Flower is that it releases the embedded emotion as well as healing the physical wound.

Healing after surgery

My thirteen-month-old baby Grace required surgery for the repair of her cleft lip. I gave her Slender Rice Flower before her surgery. The cleft lip was very noticeable, but while on this essence people began to gravitate to her as if they were drawn. All they could say was: 'How beautiful she is'. Before this, people would look away or be shocked.

It was also a godsend when surgery was performed. She needed a further procedure which normally could not have been possible until she was between four and six years old. What I realised is that there was some cooperation going on between Grace, the doctor and their spirit guides so that everything would go 'beautifully'.

Of course, I gave her Slender Rice Flower afterwards for the scarring and also with the intention of clearing any emotion associated with the scarring. Everything healed up perfectly and very quickly, even the doctors commented.

Arlene Riddick, United States

Repairing the body

A woman brought her two and a half year old adopted daughter to me. She'd been born with heart–lung problems and major surgery was due. I gave Emergency Essence to the parents, and to the child I gave:

- Waratah for her heart and to help her body respond well to surgery;
- Fringed Violet to protect her aura and to remove the effects of all she'd been through; and
- Sturt Desert Pea for her lungs.

The result was amazing. I continued to work with the little girl, and when the surgeons opened up her little body, it had repaired itself and they didn't have to do anything. Her mother says she is strong and healthy and has never looked back.

Lyn White, Western Australia

X-RAYS

If your child needs to have X-rays for any reason—for example, to check for broken bones, or at the dentist—then the remedy Mulla Mulla or the combination Solaris

Essence containing it will, if taken just beforehand and immediately afterwards, stop the body from absorbing as much of the radiation. In fact, I've received six case histories where people have taken Mulla Mulla in these circumstances and not only did the Mulla Mulla lessen the absorption of the X-rays, it totally blocked them, they couldn't obtain the X-ray. In four of the six cases the person was put on three different X-ray machines! This blocking is quite unusual—normally the result is merely less radiation in your body. Mulla Mulla is also in Travel Essence and when you are 35,000 feet above the ground in an aeroplane you absorb a lot of gamma radiation. Mulla Mulla stops the absorption and the impact of this on your body. I have read various estimates that claim an around-the-world trip involves the equivalent radiation exposure of having anywhere from four to eight chest X-rays.

Radiation

For a number of years now, my company has been donating Electro Essence to Green Cross's Radiation Rescue Program for their use in reducing levels of accumulated body radioactivity in children living in Belarus who are heavily contaminated as a direct result of the Chernobyl accident.

The results of using Electro Essence have been sensational. It reduced the children's radiation levels by 43 per cent in comparison with a control group whose levels were reduced by 3.5 per cent. This was twice as effective as the previous best treatment ever discovered by the Green Cross medical team to reduce radiation levels. What is even more astonishing is that the essence was only administered for two weeks.

One of the ancillary effects of Electro Essence was a marked reduction of many of the children's symptoms, when they physically exerted themselves, of the condition known as neurocirculatory dystonia syndrome—fainting, heart palpitations and the feeling that the heart has stopped. Electro also contributed to: the normalisation of their vegetative nervous systems; a reduced tendency to obsession; enhancement of resistance to stress; and improvement of physical and mental working capacity. Also noted were significantly fewer low-grade fevers not associated with infections; numbness of hands; and stomach ache, constipation and diarrhoea. They also complained less frequently of rapid fatigue.

Twenty-five years after the Chernobyl nuclear power plant meltdown there are still millions of people adversely affected by this disaster. This figure is likely to continue to grow as the contamination spreads further and further through the food chain and water systems. Especially vulnerable are those regions and countries in the immediate vicinity or in the direct path of the winds that carried the nuclear fallout from Chernobyl. A recent report, based on Belarus national cancer statistics, has revealed that the full consequences of the Chernobyl disaster could top 250,000 cancer cases and nearly 100,000 fatal cancers. The report concludes that radiation from the disaster has had a devastating effect on survivors; damaging immune and endocrine systems, leading to accelerated ageing, cardiovascular and blood illnesses, psychological illnesses, chromosomal aberrations and an increase in foetal deformations.

Thankfully, when society has a problem, Nature often provides a solution. Mulla Mulla, the main essence in the Electro combination, offers a safe, preventative measure to combat the increasing levels of nuclear, solar and electromagnetic radiation that we are being constantly exposed to.

Ian

Reducing household radiation

We are constantly being bombarded by electromagnetic radiation from digital phones, computers, power lines etc. By placing a bottle of Electro Essence in all four corners of your home you will greatly diminish the impact this electromagnetic radiation has on you and your family. Replace the bottles after one year.

Ian

CANCER

Fortunately, cancer* is not very common in children. Whatever the type of cancer, there needs to be a great deal of detoxifying both emotionally and physically. Purifying Essence not only works on purifying the organs of elimination but also the emotions associated with those organs: fear in the kidneys; held-on-to emotion in the large intestine; anger and resentment in the liver. Wild Potato Bush, in Purifying Essence, will also help remove heavy metals and toxic substances from the body.

If a child is having radiation therapy, then Mulla Mulla is exceptionally effective in helping minimise side effects from this treatment. For any radiation treatment for cancer, Mulla Mulla will reduce any burning, help to quickly heal any lesions that result from radiation and lessen the emotional trauma associated with radiation therapy.

If a child is given chemotherapy there can be very toxic side effects for the body, and Purifying Essence will help release the toxicity and minimise its impact on the body. Emergency Essence can be used for pain relief.

Of course, a child's reaction to the treatment and their condition can be addressed with the appropriate essences: if he is very fearful, which is understandable, Emergency Essence is excellent because it contains Grey Spider Flower, the specific remedy for terror. For children who have a fear of dying, give Bush Iris.

If your child has seen other children in the cancer ward die or they think their treatment or simply getting better is just too hard and there is a sense of giving up, then the remedy Kapok Bush would be very helpful to give them the perseverance they need. The will to live is very important when recovering from cancer, and Kapok Bush can really instil this. Some children can have a sense of 'It's not fair, why me? Why am I so sick?' Southern Cross remedy in Confid Essence will help with this attitude.

If it seems the child is going to die, then Transition Essence can ease any fear and bring a sense of calm and serenity. This essence will frequently reduce the level of morphine required, and make her passing over easier. It can give her the spiritual awareness to look for and go through the light after she dies. The remedy can be taken morning and night for up to a six-week period. It can be repeated this way as often as needed.

Transition Essence can also be taken by the rest of the family, especially siblings, to help them emotionally come to terms with their loss. It will also stop them from becoming morbid or fearful about death and dying.

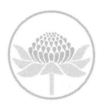

10

STARTING SCHOOL

The most significant event for children of ages five to seven is starting school. One of the best things you can do to prepare your child for school is to read regularly to him from the time he is a baby. When children are exposed to words and expression very early they are more likely to have good language and comprehension skills by the time they start school.

You can also encourage confidence and self-esteem in your child. These are the building blocks for developing independence, and confident children will always find life easier to deal with.

Also, parents need to know that simply spending time with their children, listening to them and letting them know you enjoy being with them, is how they know you care about them.

PREPARING FOR SCHOOL

Be sure to visit the school before your child starts there. Expecting a child to start at school with no preparation is like expecting an adult to start a new job with no idea of who they are going to meet, where the toilets are or what they are supposed to be doing.

Naturally, children are going to feel a little nervous about what's going to happen throughout the school day. Many schools offer opportunities for parents to bring their children along beforehand to get a sense of what is ahead. Spend time listening to your child talk about how they feel about the changes. Talk about starting school often and always in a positive way. Also, make sure that you start having morning tea and lunch at the same time as they will at school. Try to arrange some social interaction with other children starting school at the same time and going into the same class. Ensure your child has plenty of sleep in the lead up to and when starting school so they are not tired.

STARTING SCHOOL

Going off to school is a big step for little children. Many will have already been attending some form of childcare or preschool, but going to 'big' school is still a significant event.

You can help prepare your child for school by providing velcro-fastening shoes (which are easy to get on and off), pants that are easy to pull down, and also by making sure that they know basic prepositions such as in front, behind, left and right so they can follow their teacher's instructions; have had blocks and puzzles to play with as well as pencils, paints and crayons; have had opportunities to play with other children; and have had shared time when you tell each other jokes and rhymes and sing songs. All of these lay the foundations for skills in language, writing and maths, as well as physical and social skills.

However excited your child is about starting school, it can become overwhelming. After all, in that first year she will be among the smallest and youngest in a new environment, and that can be intimidating. Calm and Clear Essence is useful here because one of its remedies is Bottlebrush, which will help her through this big transition, and Paw Paw will assist if she feels overwhelmed.

IMPROVING FINE MOTOR SKILLS

Not all children have good motor coordination when they begin school. This is especially the case for boys, who on average lag behind girls by twelve months at this age. You can help prepare your child for his first year at school by making sure he can use crayons and scissors, and can button and unbutton his clothes. The remedy Bush Fuchsia will help with all motor coordination, and it will help your child distinguish between left and right.

SOCIAL IMMATURITY

Some children tend to be hyperactive and not good at social interaction. They may be quite self-focused and socially awkward and immature. Kangaroo Paw is the essence for this. Or if they are noisy and disorganised, give Jacaranda essence. Consequently, other children may shun them, making them feel isolated and lonely which can lead to attention-seeking behaviour, thus making the situation even worse.

Jacaranda essence is also very good for those children who interrupt and call out in class. They feel they need to say something while it's in their mind and so blurt out what they have to say, talking over other children and even the teacher. This can lead to them being ostracised by others and being socially isolated, which in turn can lower their self-esteem and leave the child feeling very lonely.

Starting kindergarten

I have been using Bush Flower Essences for many years and have always been passionate about their healing qualities and the wonderful results. Recently however, my son was facing some major emotional challenges dealing with trust and separation issues upon starting kindergarten. His reaction was so intense I felt there was a deeper issue he was working through, but I had no idea where to begin. I rang the Australian Bush Flower Essence Society.

To say the changes were astounding would be an understatement. Previously we both dreaded kindy days and I felt sick to the stomach watching him become more and more distressed. He has gone from screaming and shaking the gate so hard I was waiting for the fire and police departments to arrive to find out what the drama was (funny now, but not at the time) to now running up to the kindy gate, strutting in like he owns the place and asking to go to kindy on his days off. This healing was not just about kindergarten, in so many areas of his life now he is a happier, more confident and independent little boy.

There were two sets of essences used: Pink Mulla Mulla for not letting people get close; Grey Spider Flower for terror; Sydney Rose to release separation; Bottlebrush for letting go; Monga Waratah for dependence and clinginess; and Fringed Violet and Angelsword for psychic protection. Then Tall Mulla Mulla was added to the second prescription for wanting to be alone to avoid conflict.

I also sprayed my son with Purifying Essence after kindy days and regularly sprayed our home.

Lisa Constable, Queensland, Australia

Building confidence
The Bush Essence Five Corners is specific for building confidence and self-esteem. I regard it as one of the most important essences for children, and you'll find it in the combination Confid Essence.
Ian

LEARNING PROBLEMS

During these early years, children take in and need to integrate a lot of information. If your child has a learning problem, it could mean that he has retained at least some of the primitive reflexes (for more on this, see Chapter 5). When this happens, a child can easily feel overwhelmed and overloaded, and new learning will always be challenging and difficult.

There are a number of specialists working with the primitive reflexes who have found the remedy Bush Fuchsia to be the most effective treatment they've used for correcting problems associated with them.

Severe learning problems

S was recently diagnosed as having SLD (severe learning disability). He had trouble in all areas of language: speaking, memory retention (short term), comprehension, listening and stuttering as well as stumbling over words. He regularly sees a speech pathologist. Even with intensive help he can't grasp how to hold a pencil, how to draw or write letters or numbers and retain this skill for the next time.

I prescribed Bush Fuchsia and Paw Paw. Five weeks later his mother reports he has better memory retention, also when she reads to him he can often relate parts of the story to everyday life, indicating comprehension has also increased. Tall Yellow Top was added for his sense of not belonging. His mother said that he had become more vacant after moving to a new home, often walking around with a blank look on his face. Four weeks later, great news, his kindergarten teacher has remarked on his improved comprehension skills. His speech pathologist has also remarked on his improved ability in putting sentences together and using longer sentences without prompting. He is also using a larger vocabulary. S is getting less frustrated now that he has improved communication skills.

Michelle Wieber, Victoria, Australia

Breaking family patterns

A child with learning difficulties often has at least one parent who suffered similarly as a child. The remedy Boab will help to break any family pattern.
Ian

Speech enhancing

There is a little disabled boy who is the shining star of my essence work. His mother was told he would never speak, but two weeks after I prescribed

Bush Fuchsia for him, he said 'banana' and slowly continued to say more words. That was two years ago; now he is at normal school full time, has emotionally dealt with his parents' break-up and is a very together seven-year-old.

Gail Clements, Queensland, Australia

It's best to resolve learning difficulties early on where possible, because they may not improve unless addressed. Cognis Essence will strengthen all areas of learning, and one of its remedies in particular, Bush Fuchsia, will improve coordination, speech, reading and all learning skills. Bush Fuchsia is absolutely fantastic for nearly all learning problems, especially dyslexia, which can affect a child's learning, mathematics and reading. This is the specific remedy that helps to integrate the right and left hemispheres of the brain, as well as the front and back brain. If the hemispheres are not integrated when a child is reading, for example, then she will only see individual words; she won't comprehend the meaning of a sentence because all she sees is a group of words strung together.

Improving school work

Carmen and her son Sebastian had difficulty in their relationship because Sebastian never got on with his school work and everything became an endless argument. I sent Sebastian a bottle of Cognis Essence. One month later I received a letter from Carmen who said: 'Sebastian almost immediately became focused on his school work, he was more aware of the standard of work, good or bad. He rang me at work and began to cry because he had received a grade D for effort in Science. I could not believe it, as his normal behaviour was to appear not to care how he did. He revised for a task and got excellent results and was very proud of himself. He has become more able to manage his life and is far less forgetful, the result being that he is less anxious about my expectancy of him.'

Jan Brumfitt, United Kingdom

Speech difficulties

A little five-year-old boy had a learning difficulty and could only communicate with single words. The reason for this problem was unknown and his parents had taken him to many doctors and specialists, all to no avail. I suggested to his mother, my friend, that she might like to try Bush Fuchsia. Several days later she rang saying a miracle had been performed: 'almost immediately after his first dose of 7 drops, he put together the first sentence that he had ever spoken in his life!' His parents were stunned. (My husband has taken Bush Fuchsia and no longer falls asleep while reading.)

Maureen Fitchett, Australian Capital Territory

Developmental problems

Sarah, age five, has been regularly assessed by the departments of Health and Education since age six months and has been classified by them as developmentally delayed. Her parents had been advised that she would probably have to go to a special school. The reports indicated an intellectual disability, which affects her ability to communicate. She also has had difficulty processing and sorting information and her concentration and cognitive abilities have been poor. Her gross and fine motor skills were well below average, as was her coordination.

As a baby, Sarah preferred to sleep and eat small amounts. She rarely cried. As she grew older she was lethargic and showed little of the enthusiasm for life that most toddlers and preschoolers have.

After two months of Bush Fuchsia taken on and off every two weeks the parents were ecstatic about the results. Her mother wrote: 'Sarah is now very much less sleepy and is communicating well within the family. Her preschool teachers have made comment on her improvement, saying she is now making friends and communicating well in class. In a recent report, her speech therapist indicated that Sarah's speech was close to that of a "normal" child her age.

Her cognitive skills have improved and her attention span broadened, as has her ability to retain information. Next year Sarah will attend a local school and will be assisted by an aide a few hours a day. This is a long way from the school for the handicapped we had been advised a few short years ago.'
Marie Matthews, New South Wales, Australia

Some children don't integrate information when they are looking in particular directions, whether it is left, right, up or down. So if the teacher is standing in front of the class and the child is sitting on the side of the room and has to constantly look left or right to see the teacher and blackboard, she may have trouble integrating the information. The same problem can occur looking up at the blackboard or looking down when writing on paper. Children who I have treated in my clinic for learning difficulties invariably find it hard to integrate information when their eyes are looking in one of these four positions. Often they will have problems with two directions. Although simply corrected, this can cause tremendous learning difficulties for a child so afflicted. Bush Fuchsia can quickly clear this problem.

Many adults talk of overcoming their learning difficulties by developing their unique talents and skills. Businessman Richard Branson and comedian Billy Connolly are examples of people who had childhood learning difficulties that they were able to overcome or utilise to become very successful. However, they still confess that some of their problems persist in varying degrees.

Misbehaving

Ellie was a bright, happy girl, always busy. In her second year at school, she started misbehaving at school and at home. Her mother asked me to help her, so I decided to give Ellie Cognis Essence. After three days on the essence, Ellie's mother was so excited about the change in her daughter. She had slowed right down and was willing to help out in any way she could. She had also stopped being cheeky. Her teacher was amazed at the sudden change in her behaviour and her concentration in class. She was eager to learn and her reading improved.

Sue Nelson, New South Wales, Australia

When a child loses interest

If children show a tendency to become bored easily, lose interest and not finish things, this can start a pattern of behaviour that becomes a bigger problem later on. The remedy Peach-flowered Tea-tree will help these children develop drive and consistency.

Ian

LEARNING TO READ

Some children are much slower than others in learning to read. Bush Fuchsia, which is in Cognis Essence, will help with their development and, because it integrates the two hemispheres of the brain, it helps children have an understanding of what they are reading, to see the bigger picture rather than just individual words on a page that don't make sense. The Bush Fuchsia flower itself is shaped like a trumpet, and it also helps improve the clarity, tone and melody of the voice.

Inability to focus

Hugh has always been a dreamer, unable to focus on work or study. He has had a learning difficulty in that he has not been able to use right/left brain simultaneously (i.e. he could read mechanically but we gradually realised that he could not comprehend simultaneously, therefore he did not enjoy reading or studying and would not do it). After taking Bush Fuchsia things changed: he became focused, started reading and did excellently in his exams. Although the change was quick it seems to have been sustained.

Felicity Hartigan, New South Wales, Australia

Sometimes children are teased and become very embarrassed because they read so poorly in class. Fantastic results have been achieved with such children using Cognis Essence. In my Level 1 Workshops I ask for a volunteer who doesn't read very well. I then have those brave souls come to the front of the class, they are muscle tested and then I have them read out aloud from a book owned by another workshop attendee. I then retest them and invariably they test as stressed. Then I give them a dose of Bush Fuchsia and have them read a different section from the same book. The results are stunning, everyone's mouths drop because within a few seconds there is a huge difference in the volunteer's reading ability, usually going from a very incoherent monotone voice to one where there is projection, timbre, emphasis and clarity. I also ask the person what they remember after they have read both sections and often they don't remember anything from the first reading but can easily recall what they have read the second time because now it has meaning and makes sense. Consequently, they know where to put inflection rather than just reading a group of unconnected words. Frequently there are children who without Bush Fuchsia would have had to repeat a whole year of school. After the remedies they start to enjoy learning, realising they are not stupid, that they have ability, and they start improving and often excel academically.

Dyslexia

A young boy had trouble with his school work and his learning ability was poor. His teachers said he was nervous all the time in class and didn't speak up for himself. He was a very slow reader and had trouble with his words, and also tended to write letters back to front. This child had been diagnosed as having dyslexia. He had been going to classes after school to help with this but after six months there had been no change in his learning abilities. I prescribed Bush Fuchsia to help him with his poor learning abilities, and Dog Rose because his mother said he was always insecure, shy and apprehensive with other people. I saw this child three weeks later and his condition had improved a lot. He is now reading much faster and clearer and doesn't have as much trouble with his letter reversals when doing his school work. His mother said, 'He's more confident in himself and happier with himself.' He also doesn't seem so shy and insecure.

Karen A. Ballard, Australia

Boosting self-esteem

For children who have been embarrassed about their poor learning skills, it's a good idea to follow up Cognis Essence with Confid Essence to boost self-esteem.

Ian

Staying motivated and focused

My daughter Jessica is involved in programs for gifted children. I've used various essences that have helped her. For example, after taking Cognis Essence she was more settled about doing homework, going right to her work and staying until it was completed; after taking Bush Fuchsia her reading flowed better and she was eager to read and enjoyed more challenging books. Before I had to beg her to read and after she chose Sundew for herself, I noticed a quick change in her. She decided not to watch TV and was keener to do her study.

J. Parr-Elbaum, United States

THE HYPERACTIVE CHILD

If a child has a tendency towards hyperactivity*, or is obviously hyperactive, it seems to be heightened when he starts school. He has to sit in a classroom, not fidget, pay attention, and has specific work he has to do.

This is especially difficult for boys, who have testosterone acting very strongly in their bodies. This activates the large muscles, which makes them more physically active and they need to run around, using up energy. Because a boy's fine motor coordination develops later than it does in girls, little boys often feel inferior to the girls in the class. They feel frustrated that they aren't as skilled, become bored and play up. When they are made to sit still and pay attention they can become frustrated and disruptive.

Hyperactive children need to have short, clear, precise instructions, otherwise they become overwhelmed and overloaded. Cognis Essence is the main combination for the hyperactive child. It includes these remedies:

- Jacaranda, which helps your child if he is easily distracted;
- Bush Fuchsia, which integrates the left and right hemispheres of the brain and helps with hearing;
- Paw Paw, which helps your child take in information;
- Sundew, which assists with attention to detail; and
- Isopogon, for enhancing memory.

Severe dyslexia

Liam, a seven-year-old boy, suffers from severe dyslexia, a family problem. Already after two weeks of taking Bush Fuchsia essence his mother noticed a complete change in the way Liam reads, writes and expresses himself.
Louise Tuyt-Snippe, The Netherlands

Attention deficit hyperactivity disorder (ADHD)

There are nine times as many boys diagnosed with attention deficit hyperactivity disorder* as there are girls and Ritalin is widely prescribed for this condition. In my state, New South Wales, 1 in 36 latter primary school-aged children are being given this drug. Diagnosis of ADHD and ADD is difficult and not uniform and is often criticised for the frequency of misdiagnosis. However, it is estimated that between 2 and 6 per cent of children show the key symptoms of hyperactivity, impulsiveness and inattentiveness, though it is frequent that girls fail to be identified and boys are wrongly labelled and treated.

The great concern is whether Ritalin is a quick medical fix that replaces any attempt to determine the underlying causes. Many boys struggle with basic literacy for a wide range of reasons and this has been put down as one of the reasons why they are so disruptive and then subsequently labelled with ADHD. For many boys the school system is very basic and ill-suited to their needs. As well as the influence of testosterone, discussed earier, boys are not as developmentally mature as girls. As mentioned, they may have greater difficulty with tasks such as writing, cutting and sewing when compared to girls, which can lead to further frustration ending in disruptive behaviour leading to their diagnosis.

Research is showing that behaviour labelled as ADHD may simply be a response to the way a child has been taught. Many boys have difficulty with the high level of verbal reasoning and written communication skills required by the current curriculum, and it is often beyond their developmental capacity. Up to 20 per cent of six-year-old boys cannot process verbal information beyond an eight-word sentence. So if teachers are giving verbal instructions using sentences longer than that, a proportion of the children will lose much of the detail of what they have been told and can start acting out and getting into trouble.

Studies have shown that merely having the teachers slow down their instructions, use shorter sentences, maintain eye contact and wait for compliance can greatly improve a child's learning progress and behaviour, especially for boys. When boys have been able to improve their literacy, their behaviour in class has improved dramatically. Again, remedies such as Bush Fuchsia can be utilised to improve reading and literacy.

It has been found that between 70 and 85 per cent of children assessed as being at risk of underachievement are boys. There has been criticism that the school curriculum needs to be made more relevant for boys. Older, more experienced teachers are also complaining that recently graduated teachers often encourage parents to medicate their children to calm down disruptive boys while ignoring any social problems that might be occurring in the home life of these children. Boys are often unable to express feelings about problems at home such as domestic violence, divorce or separation, and often become inattentive, rude and disruptive far more so than girls, and of course they can then be labelled ADHD.

Amazing change

I recently had an amazing case. A six-year-old boy had been diagnosed as having ADHD, Asperger's syndrome, eating disorders, learning and speaking problems–the lot. His behaviour was outrageous: he put his younger brother in hospital several times! He had slept only three or four hours out of every 24 from the time he was a baby. He had been assessed at school as being mid-preschool standard and he had no social skills. He wouldn't go out of the house unless forced and fought violently with any kids he did get to play with. He made life hell for everyone. I gave him a mix of Fringed Violet, Sundew, Bush Fuchsia, Crowea, Dog Rose, Macrocarpa and Kangaroo Paw. From the sixth day after starting the mix there was marked improvement. He willingly went to visit his grandmother and allowed her to give him a hug–something he had never done before. And on the same day his speech teacher commented that for the first time since she had been working with him he was actually listening and responding. By the time the next school year started he was reassessed and found to be middle of the range for his age at reading and comprehension. His new teacher didn't even know he had any problems. His mother said to me, 'I feel for the first time since he was born that I have a normal child!'

Marie Matthews, New South Wales, Australia

There is a school of thought among psychologists and child educationists that social and environmental changes create disturbances in the child's capacity for self-regulation. This may explain why so many children are unable to accept or follow instructions and show high levels of acting out behaviour associated with learning problems. One of the biggest stress factors for children affecting both their self-regulation and attentiveness is the decrease in quality time for infants and young children with their parents or caretakers, parents being under greater time pressures than ever before. This, coupled with longer periods in poor-quality childcare together with divorce and the absence of fathers, forms the emotional foundation that interacts with and contributes to neurological function. Certainly, I have found in my clinic that learning goes down as stress goes up. Giving Bush Fuchsia is very specific for treating any neuro-developmental disorders, together with Paw Paw for any feeling of being overwhelmed. It has also been noticed that boys will cover up their vulnerability when trying to make emotional contact through disruptive behaviour. It is often interpreted as aggressive both by parents and teachers. Wisteria, Flannel Flower and Bluebell will all help these problems. Certainly it is the boys who are far more prone to be disruptive in their behaviour when there are family break-ups and perform badly at school in response to long hours in childcare.

Behavioural problems

Dennis, aged five, presented with severe behavioural problems and irrational outbursts. He was withdrawn, showing poor learning, having nightmares and sleeping in Mum's bed, and displayed a lack of coordination. A decision had been made that Dennis would not be progressing to a higher grade next year. His mother and father separated two years ago and he lives with his mother, who works, and he is cared for by his grandmother. Visits with his father are infrequent and often cancelled. Through kinesiology it was ascertained that right and left brains were not integrated.

I prescribed Bush Fuchsia and Grey Spider Flower. Two weeks later his mother said the school had approached her stating his behaviour had improved dramatically, his concentration was better and he was not such a destructive influence. Dennis reports that the teacher likes him better and even Mum does too.

Bush Fuchsia and Grey Spider Flower continued for another two weeks and on the third visit his moods were fluctuating little and he was now sleeping in his own bed and finding it easy to get up in the morning. His teacher is amazed how his work is improving. Red Helmet Orchid was added to the two other remedies and at the next visit his mum said his moods had settled and he was calmer, school work was still improving and the teacher said he is a delightful child.

(Name supplied but withheld on request)

There are certainly children who have a problem with paying attention, sitting still and who will be noisy and impulsive. Black-eyed Susan, found in Calm and Clear Essence, will help settle and calm them down, making them less impatient. Jacaranda, a remedy in Cognis Essence (which is the main combination for the hyperactive child), will assist them to stay focused on something for a period of time. Normally such children are easily distracted, so if the classroom is noisy they may be having trouble learning as they won't be able to focus very well and their minds will start wandering. Another area Jacaranda can assist with is impulsiveness, helping them to think before acting so that they don't have a knee-jerk reaction to what is going on around them. Sundew, also in Cognis Essence, can be used when children are being too dreamy and vague, disorganised, having trouble concentrating, following plans or keeping things tidy. It is a very grounding, earthing remedy aiding attention to detail.

Often children with ADHD will have problems with sleeping. They become easily excited and find it difficult to calm down enough to go to bed. Calm and Clear Essence will calm them down and prepare them for sleep. Spray it in the bedroom and apply the cream to the child's hands and face. Playing the White Light CD will also help to calm them. The music will help your child settle down so they can drift off to sleep. This CD will also have them waking more energised and less grumpy.

Helping ADHD

I have a nine-year-old son who has been diagnosed with ADHD. He is very psychic and hyperactive and has severe learning and behavioural problems, poor digestion etc. He fits the pattern of an indigo child. He needs to get his message across and will keep pushing and hounding people until he knows they understand. Over the years I have tried many things to help him. But when I recently tried the Bush Essences Cognis and Kangaroo Paw there was a complete turn around. He is not so much in your face, and he wants to go to school instead of the teacher virtually having to drag him into the classroom. He wants to learn and his handwriting has improved dramatically from being indecipherable to being very clear and readable.

Danielle Muir, New South Wales, Australia

Aiding social skills
Children who are hyperactive are often unaware of others and their needs. The remedy Kangaroo Paw will help them with this and it is the specific remedy for poor social skills.
Ian

In 1995 the US Drug Enforcement Agency expressed grave concerns about Ritalin because 'it shares many of the pharmacological effects of . . . cocaine'. I've had many patients who've said that when they were put on to Ritalin they felt that their emotional development stopped, as if they were cut off from their feelings. Cognis Essence is a much more effective treatment and has absolutely no side effects. Studies in the United States have shown a correlation between Ritalin use in childhood and cocaine and amphetamine use in adulthood. I find the results from Cognis Essence are far superior to Ritalin, and totally safe.

Ritalin alternative
Bonnie Wisnewskiski from Hong Kong, whose son had been on Ritalin for attention deficit syndrome, said she had never felt comfortable with this treatment. Cognis Essence was recommended to her, and she reports, 'I have seen very encouraging results and am so happy to have my son off the Ritalin. He seems so much more himself and he is now enjoying school a great deal.'
Ian

THE IMPORTANCE OF PLAY

Some parents think that once children start school, the days of playing are over. But children need plenty of opportunities to play both before they start school and throughout childhood. In fact, the time to play and imagine and dream continues to be important throughout life, and most adults would be much healthier and calmer if they took time out to play. Little Flannel Flower is the essence that addresses the expression of playfulness and being carefree. It is excellent for children who tend to grow up too quickly, taking on the troubles of the world and becoming old before their time.

MAKING FRIENDS

It is helpful to children if they start school knowing a few other children in the class. Research shows that children who start off with friends at school and continue to make new friends will be happier at school. All the same, some children are more solitary than others and prefer their own company. It's up to parents to be sensitive to their child's needs and not to push friendships on to them.

Children are more likely to make friends easily when they have a healthy self-esteem. Confid Essence is excellent here. Its remedy Five Corners raises self-esteem and increases self-love, and its remedy Dog Rose builds courage and confidence, especially for a shy child.

Poor bonding

If you and your child did not bond early, you could find that your child tends to be separate and alone in his relationships. He may find it difficult to make friends, and shy away from other children even when they try to include him in games. Some children tend to be natural loners and are often good observers. They are happy to be on the outside of groups but they do have good interaction skills. But there are some children who simply don't know how to interact, and this can cause difficulties throughout their schooling and may continue into adulthood. The remedy Tall Yellow Top is very good in this case because it addresses the sense of loneliness and isolation and gives a feeling of belonging. It will also give your child the valuable ability to reach out to others.

BEING BULLIED

If your child suddenly doesn't like going to school or is trying to avoid it, or her school work has suddenly deteriorated and she is generally unhappy, one possible explanation is that she is being bullied. There are other warning signs too, such as becoming withdrawn, being aggressive with siblings or having nightmares*. Sometimes it's the child who has low self-esteem and is more isolated socially who is more likely to be picked on. If this is the case, Kangaroo Paw will help them to achieve better social interaction with the rest of the children in the class, while Confid Essence will help their self-esteem and address any anxiety, a common consequence of being bullied. A recent study from the University of Western Sydney shows that playground bullying can cause the same level of psychological trauma as child abuse. Certainly higher levels of depression, suicidal thoughts and attempts at self-harm often occur in children who are bullied. Waratah, in Emergency Essence, is specific to help with these symptoms. There are some very disturbing statistics associated with bullying in Australian primary schools. Fifteen per cent of students have experienced cyber-bullying with text messages or information about them being placed on the internet. Fifty per cent of students have experienced face-to-face (which is the nastier) bullying at least once in the last term, while 20 per cent experienced it in the last week or more, bearing in mind that bullying is often unreported. The name of an older child can be Googled to see if they are being bullied on the net. Of course, the problem with technology is that bullying can occur 24 hours a day where previously it was only on the way to and from, or at, school. Sometimes, too, a child can feel ineffective and hopeless in these situations and Kapok Bush addresses that sense of just wanting to give up.

Children who tend to be loners can also be picked on because there is less chance of friends sticking up for them. Both Pink and Tall Mulla Mulla are remedies for loners. Tall Yellow Top is the remedy for children who feel isolated, who are not part of groups and are lonely. These are key targets for bullies.

There are more reports of bullying by primary school students than high school students. Boys are more likely to experience direct physical bullying where girls are more likely to be victims of indirect non-physical forms of bullying such as exclusion and rumours being spread about them. Direct verbal bullying, teasing etc., is the most common form of bullying in children and affects boys and girls equally.

Confid Essence gives the child being bullied the courage to stand up to and confront the bully; it gives them strength of character to stand their ground, which invariably makes the bully back away.

As mentioned, bullying can be very traumatic for children and if not addressed can lead to a lot of pain and suffering for them at the time but can also have deeper ramifications later in life. There are some very disturbing statistics around young people today: more than 1 in 5 has a mental health problem, including adolescents. Ten per cent of eighteen to 25 year olds will experience anxiety within any 12-month period. Mental health problems can begin in children as young as five. Depression and anxiety are two of the most common mental health issues accounted by adolescents but if there is childhood bullying this could be a trigger for developing depression and anxiety later in adolescence. For depression there are three remedies in particular: Tall Yellow Top, Waratah and Pink Flannel Flower. It is important, too, to work with Emergency Essence to address initial trauma. It is well recognised that untreated mental disorders often develop into more complex conditions later in adolescence. Bush Essences offer a very effective tool for dealing with issues like anxiety and depression. It can be very healing but also preventive against further problems later in life.

The bullied child

Fringed Violet, in Emergency Essence, is another remedy that can help a bullied child, providing some psychic protection around them.
Ian

Being a bully

For a child who is doing the bullying, the remedy Rough Bluebell will help her develop empathy and compassion. It is empathy that for most people nips in the bud the desire to direct anger or frustration towards others, including children. Seeing another person unhappy or hurt elicits an empathic response. But for real bullies other people's hurt doesn't touch them, and this is where Rough Bluebell is so helpful. Usually bullies don't feel good about themselves; they can experience a lot of low self-esteem, so Confid Essence is good for them too.

Also, many psychologists report that the bullies they treat often have a lot of guilt about what they are doing and have nowhere to go and feel bad about being a bully. Sturt Desert Rose is for guilt and is also in Confid Essence. Often being a bully is a mask they put on to hide their own vulnerability.

Many bullies come from emotionally or physically abusive home environments so Sexuality Essence and Emergency Essence would be beneficial for them. These children will often feel powerless or helpless at home, due to conflict between the parents or the violence and abuse they receive at home, and this in turn leads them to choose vulnerable targets because it allows them to experience a sense of power over someone.

It is often hard for parents to notice that their child is a bully. If there are reports of your child bullying they need to be taken seriously. They should be made to give back anything they have taken (toys or money), and attention should not be focused on them—this is often what they are seeking so make sure the behaviour is not reinforced. They also need to be made to apologise to the person they have bullied and punishments put in place. Bullies are rewarded if there is no intervention and they get attention from their peers. Peer mediation between the two students, and a neutral student monitoring conversations, is something that is proving to be very effective in a lot of primary schools as well as high schools. If there is a family history of domination, bullying or aggression, then Boab can be given to the child to help break that cycle. Gymea Lily also may be a constitution remedy for children who are natural leaders but who are often very bossy and tend to use their natural charisma and power to dominate weaker children.

Child bullies invariably grow up to be adult bullies; it is good if their behaviour can be modified early.

WHEN DAD IS ABSENT

If your child's father is not present, perhaps because he spends long hours at work, you have separated or he has died, then the bond between you and your child can be very intense. You may find yourself playing the role of father as well as mother, and this can be confusing for both you and your child.

You can help bring more balance to the relationship between you and your child by giving him Red Helmet Orchid. This is the remedy for unresolved father issues, which can show up in rebellious attitudes to anyone in authority such as teachers.

STILL BEDWETTING

About 10 per cent of children starting kindergarten are still bedwetting* at night. If this continues it can cause real problems for children, especially when they start being asked to have sleepovers with friends.

The kidney relates to fear in Chinese medicine, and Dog Rose is the remedy that addresses this. It is the main remedy for bedwetting. I've also found that adding Red Helmet Orchid, the remedy that relates to the father, is a brilliant solution.

Bedwetting

A six-year-old boy who was bedwetting frequently was distressed about it. His mother came to me for help. I chose Grey Spider Flower for fears, terror and nightmares, as bedwetting is a symptom of fear. This essence is also related to kidneys, which are the seat of fear. I sensed there could have been an element of psychic attack involved, possibly with the astral body splitting from the causal during sleep, and this essence would help with this. I also gave him Billy Goat Plum because of the shame the boy had developed around the bedwetting. It led him to distrust his body, especially his urinary system. This essence would help him accept his physical self and release shame and guilt.

After two nights the bedwetting ceased and stayed clear. He and his mother were very excited about the results.

Christine Flynn, New South Wales, Australia

Sometimes the child feels anxious, perhaps about the father but possibly regarding some other authority figure like a teacher. We've had many case histories where Bush Essences have resolved the problem. In one story from South America, the father had spent thousands of dollars flying his seven-year-old son from Brazil to the United States for special treatment for bedwetting, all to no avail. The father was a very successful businessman, very abrupt and not very sensitive, and his son was fearful around him. Once the child took Dog Rose and Red Helmet Orchid, the anxiety disappeared and the bedwetting stopped. When all this was explained to the father, he asked if there were essences he could take to help him become more sensitive and less intimidating to his son.

A FUSSY EATER

Sometimes a child is considered a fussy eater when she avoids intuitively things she knows she has a sensitivity or allergy* to. She may not want to eat foods that contain certain natural or artificial chemicals. Pay attention to what your child may not want to eat.

A child who is resistant to change may also be a fussy eater. She is not interested in anything that's different or unusual to her. The remedy Freshwater Mangrove is for a child who has already made up her mind about a food without even trying it, and the remedy Bauhinia is to help her be open to something a bit different or something she is not used to eating.

When a child is not eating much this may be because she doesn't have good digestion; a combination of Paw Paw and Crowea will help stimulate the appetite and help digestion as well. If this is a family pattern, try adding Boab to the other two essences.

For parents: Your child's eating habits
If you feel distressed about your child's eating habits, Crowea, which is in both Emergency Essence and Calm and Clear Essence, will address the worrying and help to calm you down. Sometimes children react to their parents' worry and fussing. When you are calmer and less worried about whether your child is eating enough, she may become more interested in food.
Ian

OBESITY

There is an obesity epidemic affecting nearly every developed country in the world today. It is affecting both children and adults. Fat children invariably end up as fat adults. In Australia there have been some alarming changes in just one generation: 20 per cent of boys and 24 per cent of girls in New South Wales aged from five to sixteen are overweight or obese compared with only 11 per cent of all young people aged seven to sixteen just 25 years ago. In the United States 20 to 40 per cent of under ten year olds are overweight or obese. One's quality of life is certainly affected by being overweight and obese. These children are highly likely to develop type 2 diabetes later in life and run the risk of developing problems with high blood pressure, cardiovascular disease as well as orthopaedic problems as they get older. There has been a vast amount of research focused on possible links between genes, hormones and obesity. But the bottom line is that obesity is not due to genetics—it is due to environment and the food being consumed. If you eat more food than you expend in energy, you are going to put on weight.

High-fat foods have twice the energy of either sugar or proteins. Fat also does not suppress appetite as well as the other two food groups and especially protein. So even small amounts of food, if they are high in fat, can lead to weight gain.

In European studies it has been found that the Dutch have a very similar diet to their neighbours the Germans and also to the British, yet they have much lower obesity levels. The main reason put down for this was that 70 per cent of journeys to and from work in The Netherlands are done by pushbike as opposed to only 10 per cent in the United Kingdom.

Overweight children need to be more physically active than they are now. Unfortunately many parents are often reluctant, due to safety issues, to let their children run around and play outside. Consequently many children are spending too much time playing video games and watching TV, which have been shown to lead to obesity and being overweight. Primarily the problem is that these activities are low in calorie expenditure and the children are exposed to junk food advertising which influences what they want to eat. Also, children are more likely to snack in front of the TV and studies have shown that children will overeat by up to 20 per cent if eating meals in front of the TV rather than if they are sitting around the dinner table.

To help break the TV habit, studies overseas have shown that success can be achieved by first determining how much TV is being watched by a child, then seeing if your child will recognise that as too much. Have him compare it to how much his peers are watching. Then make a list of what he really likes to watch. Limit the TV time to only what he wishes to watch. Have a ten-day period when there is no TV. This can help break a whole lot of habits. Wonderful things have happened in this time; children have found new friends living nearby to go out and play with. Then restrict viewing to seven hours a week and no eating while watching TV.

Flannel Flower is an essence to help children be more motivated to physically express themselves and be active. Bush Fuchsia works on the hypothalamus, which controls the appetite centre.

If there are bad eating habits in the family, Boab can be used to help break those patterns. Bottlebrush and Boronia help break habits of snacking between meals and eating food that is not nourishing. Drinking more water will suppress the appetite, so encourage your children to drink a glass of water rather than reaching for food in between meals. Other essences that can be useful are Monga Waratah to help with willpower and for not eating junk food and Hibbertia for developing good eating disciplines.

Dagger Hakea harmonises the gall bladder, the organ necessary for effective digestion of fatty foods. On the issue of fat, in a recent study in the United States a high fat diet of potato chips, peanut butter and chocolate was given to pregnant monkeys whose foetuses were then found to develop fatty liver disease, a potential precursor to diabetes. It did not matter whether the adult monkeys who ate the high-fat diet got fat themselves. The fact they were eating that food led to the fatty liver problems in the foetus and all the baby monkeys had fatty livers too. Researchers saw this as an indication that fat in the diet when they were in the womb made the offspring more likely to become obese. It implicated saturated fat in the diet as the culprit.

Fatty liver disease is now becoming more common in young children, where previously it was only seen in patients who were obese for many years in adult life. Some studies estimate that half of all obese children have fatty liver problems, which can also lead to liver failure.

Diabetes

A three-year-old girl came for healing. She had been diagnosed with diabetes at 22 months and was having three injections of insulin daily. Her abdomen was swollen from the insulin. I prescribed Peach-flowered Tea-tree for the diabetes and to instil a sense of taking responsibility for her illness. The mother was constantly assessing her, and so the disease was given a lot of power.

I also prescribed Fringed Violet to keep her aura intact and to protect her from psychic attack.

A few weeks later there seemed to be some improvement. The mother was pleased with the results. By the next visit the insulin had been reduced. The little girl continued to improve not needing insulin every day, sometimes only every third day! She learnt to love her pancreas. When the mother took her daughter to the paediatrician who I was working in conjunction with, he said there was a remarkable difference in her condition and to continue the drops.

Pam Knights, New South Wales, Australia

FOOD INTOLERANCE

There is a difference between an allergy to a food and a food intolerance*. An allergy involves the immune system and the reaction is usually immediate, whereas food intolerance involves an irritation to nerve endings in various parts of the body. Usually there is not the immediate reaction that there is with allergies, and sometimes a food intolerance can build up over time.

If a child has an intolerance to a particular food, they may be able to tolerate a small amount of that food with no symptoms. However, if they have an allergy to a food even the smallest amount can cause problems.

Some of the more common intolerances are to natural substances, such as salicylates, amines and glutamates. Many fruits contain salicylates, such as berries, oranges and grapes, and they are also present in high quantities in some nuts, spices, jam and honey. High amounts of glutamates are found in ripe tomatoes, cheese, mushrooms, meat and yeast extracts. Fermented foods are high in amines. Preservatives in foods are another common cause of food intolerance.

When children are very young, food intolerances tend to show up in the form of skin rashes*, colic* or sleeping problems*. As they grow into the toddler phase they can suffer breathing difficulties, diarrhoea, tantrums*, anxiety* and general behavioural problems. If one or both parents, or other children in the family, have similar symptoms, then Boab will help clear any family patterns.

Medical studies in this area are not common, but a recent UK study found a definite link between food colourings and hyperactivity*. The study showed that a food intolerance would worsen any already existing hyperactivity in a child.

The first place of good digestion is in the mouth, and if eating is rushed the result can be an allergic reaction. Gulping down food without chewing it properly means the body may interpret poorly digested protein molecules in the stomach as foreign matter if this frequently occurs. The result is that the allergic surveillance mast cells attach and release histamines to cope with the proteins.

After it leaves the stomach the food goes to the small intestine, where the fats and carbohydrates are further broken down. Dagger Hakea will work on the gall bladder and the bile, and Peach-flowered Tea-tree will help with the proper absorption of nutrients in the small intestine. Food leaves the small intestine via the ileocaecal valve and enters the large intestine. The remedy Bauhinia will help with good functioning of the ileocaecal valve. If this valve is blocked then everything starts to accumulate and the contents of the small intestine start to ferment. If the valve is leaky you get backflow from the large intestine into the small intestine. The two intestines have different pH levels and different bacteria, so backflow can cause many problems including headaches, digestive problems as well as allergies and food intolerances.

A common approach to food intolerance is to introduce a rotational diet. This involves sorting food into categories and rotating them so, for example, eggs and poultry are eaten only once every four days, dairy once every four days, wheat once every four days. By rotating the food families once every four days, it is easier to pick up on what your child may be sensitive to. Notice what your child was eating on the day she complained of a tummy ache or a runny nose or a headache, or when she was slightly aggressive or had trouble concentrating.

In numerology, if a child is born with the numbers 7, 8 and 9 all in their birth date they will have a greater susceptibility to colourings and additives in the food. Generally children shouldn't be eating these, or very sugary or refined foods. All these foods can have an adverse effect on their behaviour.

NAIL BITING MOMENTS

Some children chew away at their nails until there's little left of them. Some nibble away just a little. Nail biting is one of the most common of children's habits and in most cases they grow out of it.

It could be that your child is biting her nails out of anxiety*. If you think this is the case the remedy Crowea will settle nerves and bring peace and calm. You'll find Crowea in Emergency Essence and also Calm and Clear Essence. At the same time you could suggest some alternatives to nail biting: keeping fingers busy by drawing, or playing shadow puppets. This will distract your child from the nail biting so that she's more likely to consider other, more constructive activities.

IF YOUR CHILD IS OUT OF SORTS

From time to time your child might appear to be flat, out of sorts* or not quite right. It could be due to a number of factors: your child could have a mild illness, or could be suffering from constipation*. Whatever the case, Crowea is the general remedy for re-establishing balance. It works as a general tonic for the organs and the meridians in the body. It is in both Emergency Essence and Calm and Clear Essence.

Physical weakness

A girl was brought to me who was pale and listless. She had been prescribed many antibiotics over the years and so she had missed a lot of schooling. She hadn't spent a full week at school for almost a year. She was a bright and willing student, but was physically weak and prone to bad ear infections. Her mother was told that an operation was 'the best bet' after yet another infection, but the mother turned to me. Among the essences I prescribed were:

- Red Grevillea for infection;
- Bush Fuchsia for the ears; and
- Illawarra Flame Tree to support her immune system and feeling of rejection for her brother who had been receiving a lot of attention.

Within days she was recovering. Three weeks later there was no sign of illness, she had her first week without missing school, she was completely different, plucky, confident and more balanced, and she had signed up for gymnastic classes!

Trudi Nichols, United Kingdom

THE SCOURGE OF HEAD LICE

Head lice* are tiny parasites that are spread by having head-to-head contact with someone else who has them. They are very common in children, especially when they start school. Having clean hair is no guarantee that your child will not suffer head lice. The favourite place for lice to feed is on the scalp behind the ears and at the nape of the neck. Their sucking action is what causes the main symptom of lice—scratching.

To treat head lice, cover your child's hair with conditioner and comb carefully, strand by strand, with a fine-toothed comb. Black-eyed Susan can be given to a child before you start to allow them to sit still and be patient for a long while, especially if they have long hair. Dispose of the conditioner containing the lice and their eggs. Give your child Green Essence drops internally as well as spraying it on the hair, the remedy for any parasite on or in the body. Billy Goat Plum is for any feelings of being dirty or unclean, together with shame and embarrassment about having nits, especially if their friends at school know.

GRIEF AND BEREAVEMENT

If someone in the family is dying, whether it's a parent, sibling or grandparent, all the family will be affected and have issues around death. Transition Essence is useful for everyone concerned. It helps everyone cope and move through any major life change. It eases the fear of death while helping you come to terms with it. A great deal of feelings and emotions can come up for a child experiencing bereavement. There can be anger, resentment, grief, even guilt and resignation. It is important that children are allowed to express what they are feeling.

The remedy Bluebell helps a child get in touch with their feelings, especially when there are a lot of them and many they have not felt before. Crowea is used when there is a great intensity of emotion, while Flannel Flower can help them to talk about and express what it is they are feeling. Counsellors often recommend gently bringing up the subject but waiting until the child is ready to discuss and then be able to answer questions. Quite often younger children will have a lot of questions they will repeat over and over until they get it clearly in their mind. Death can often lead to younger children feeling guilt because they are so egocentric they think they are responsible for the death, and it needs to be explained that nobody is to blame. If there are feelings of guilt then Sturt Desert Rose in Confid Essence can be very healing.

For the initial rawness of emotion on hearing the news or seeing it, Red Suva Frangipani is very good. Some children can even go backwards in their development in response to grief. Maintaining routines is very good, having meals at the same time, for example, so they realise that life carries on even though there is a lot of sadness. Some children can be very withdrawn (in which case use Kapok Bush) or they can become hyperactive, filling their time with activity to stop the uncomfortable feelings—use Black-eyed Susan here.

Unlike adults, children are likely to move in and out of grief quite quickly; sometimes they are still suffering when they are experiencing grief. Some children get very confused with sudden turnarounds. It is reassuring to let them know it's okay to have love and laughter back in their life even though there are some times when there is sadness as well. Little Flannel Flower can be a very good remedy to keep their playfulness present. Pink Flannel Flower will ease some of the burden and pain in their hearts to stop them getting too miserable and sad.

Many children are very sensitive to the feelings of others, especially today's children. They will pick up on the grief* and sadness that others in the family are feeling, especially if it is their parent who is losing one of their own parents. The remedy Fringed Violet, in Emergency Essence, will help because it will give a child psychic protection from other people's pain and suffering.

I've found that some children have an air of grief and sadness about them for much of the time, yet their parents can't think of any specific reason for this. A lot of research has now revealed that it is not uncommon for people to have a twin in the womb who does not survive. The surviving twin can be left with a degree of sadness and grief on a deep psychological level. Wherever there is sadness in the personality, think of Sturt Desert Pea, which releases deeply held grief and sadness. This remedy works extremely quickly in almost all cases, even when the pain has been harboured for many years, even as far back as a previous life.

Fear and grief

A boy was brought to me after his father passed over from cancer. He was a quiet, introverted boy who had become very fearful and indecisive. His mother wanted to help him cope with fear and grief. The main essence I prescribed was Dog Rose for worry, shyness, insecurity and unresolved grief (which in Chinese medicine can trigger fear and anxiety). There was a noticeable change in the boy at his second consultation, he appeared lighter, open with more smiles. This time I prescribed Sturt Desert Pea for the grief of losing his father, and Red Suva Frangipani to deal with the raw emotions associated with grief and loss. He seemed much more secure when I next saw him, and gave a lot more eye contact.

Wendy Driscoll, New South Wales, Australia

Regaining innocence

A little boy, in a case where a father dies, or alternatively a little girl if her mother dies, often grows up quite quickly and, if he is the oldest child, takes on the mantle of being the man of the house (or the woman of the house). In these situations the children lose their innocence and childhood under that burden of responsibility. Little Flannel Flower can help them stay childlike, innocent and playful once they have dealt with the initial shock and gone through the initial grieving period for the loss of their parent. This of course can also occur when there is separation through divorce.

Ian

SEPARATION OR DIVORCE

If there has been a divorce, one of the important things is reassuring children they are loved. Because they are so egocentric, young children often blame themselves for the separation or divorce* of their parents. They think they are responsible because they didn't pick up their toys, or they didn't go to bed earlier or they had a tantrum.

Sadly, twelve months after a separation, around 30 per cent of men have not had contact with their children. It can be heartbreaking for the father and devastating for the child, who may feel abandoned. The remedy Red Helmet Orchid will help here, resolving father issues and strengthening the bond between father and child even when the father is not around.

If it's the mother who is not seeing her child after a separation, then Bottlebrush will help both her and her child to strengthen that bond between them.

Divorce can bring huge upheaval to a family. It may mean moving house, or moving to a new neighbourhood and a new school among other changes. Bottlebrush helps here because it makes any change that much easier to handle. This was the essence given to six-year-old Sebastian when his parents divorced. His practitioner, Natasha Fernandez of Uruguay, prescribed it for him not only because of the major changes in his life, but to strengthen the bond with his mother. She also prescribed Red Helmet Orchid because he was having serious problems with his dad. As well, she gave him Dagger Hakea so that he could more openly express the anger he was bottling up, and Fringed Violet to protect him from the negative energy of the situation. 'The first change in Sebastian was that he began to express his feeling of anger to his parents,' she wrote. 'His behaviour started to change positively at school, and he left behind his violent attitude.'

Of course behaviour changes can be very common in children as a result of divorce or even the death of a parent. Their behaviour in school can quite often be disruptive or they can become very quiet and withdrawn. Teachers need to be aware of what is happening in their home situation. Their concentration can be very distracted and they can't focus. Cognis Essence addresses both of these issues. Sometimes they will be more vague and dreamy, splitting off and being out of their bodies because what is happening in their world is too painful for them. There may be a lot of anger and resentment, and Dagger Hakea can be very useful if they perceive the changes in their world to be their parents' faults.

159

Another aspect of divorce is that it is quite often a precursor to a child living in a step-family situation, maybe not initially but down the track. The parent they live with may later become involved with a partner who has children themselves, so they may from a brand new family unit, which can be very stressful. Second marriages have a much higher rate of divorce than first marriages because there is a lot more baggage being brought in. About 50 per cent of second marriages where there are other children involved will eventually end in divorce, and a total of around 25 per cent of these step-families break up within their first year. The remedies for change such as Bottlebrush and Bauhinia will be useful if such changes are to occur—Bottlebrush for when the change is happening, Bauhinia to help introduce the idea to the young child of the new family dynamic that will be occurring.

Dealing with divorce

Tashy was six years old when her parents separated and she would wail 'It's not fair. How come you're separating and no other Mums and Dads are?' After taking Southern Cross, the remedy for anyone who feels hard done by, Tashy settled remarkably well. She was far less reactive and miserable.

She seemed guilty all the time when her parents separated. She kept saying 'sorry' as though she was to blame. I gave her Sturt Desert Rose to dissolve the feeling of guilt.

Rachel, address withheld on request

For blended families it can be very useful for the parents to spray the remedy Slender Rice Flower around the house, to bring about group harmony. Another remedy is Sturt Desert Rose. If the parent with whom the child lives has a new partner, sometimes the child can feel she is being disloyal to her other parent if she is close, friendly and loving to the new person. It can be a very difficult time for a child. Fortunately, children have a lot of emotional flexibility, even more so than their parents, and are quite resilient through such major changes. As a result of divorce some children become very clingy, having the sense of losing one parent, so they hold on more to the one they are living with. Consider Monga Waratah for over-dependence as well as Dog Rose for anxiety and Illawarra Flame Tree for the fear of being rejected. All these remedies can help reduce the clinginess seen in divorce or with the death of a parent.

For a child who is used to one set of rules, then suddenly has a step-parent and has to adjust to brand new rules and regulations, there can be a lot of jealousy and not wanting to share their parent with another person. Mountain Devil is the remedy for jealousy. There is one other remedy, Mint Bush, to use when it feels as if everything is in perturbation, with change and chaos in their world; this remedy can help settle things.

Turning a negative into a positive

My two daughters spend 50 per cent of time at their father's place where there is a lot of stress and tension and negativity. When they return they are always grumpy and very badly behaved. Recently I have been spraying the girls and their bags and anything that they have brought from their dad's with Space Clearing room spray. Within ten to fifteen minutes both girls are lovely, well behaved and happy. It's like a mini-miracle! And I feel totally supported and therefore have a much more relaxed approach to any potentially lethal situation—I can always use the 'spray' to turn negativity into positivity.

(Name supplied but withheld on request)

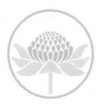

11

KNOWING YOUR CHILD

When I first started studying naturopathy I also undertook a course in numerology, an ancient system used to determine a person's life path and give insights into their personality. I learnt the Pythagorean system of numerology, which I found to be an invaluable tool. It is very quick, accurate, easy to use and provides a great insight into the personality of a person. I have been practising naturopathy for over thirty years, and I have done the numerology chart of every patient I have ever treated.

In young children born since the year 2000, we are now seeing unusual patterns that in some cases haven't been seen for over one thousand years. In my clinical experience I've found that by doing a child's numerology chart—even when they are very young, before they can talk—you can pinpoint specific strengths they have as well as challenges they will face. In this chapter I'll suggest specific Bush Essences you can use to enhance your child's strengths. As your child grows, you can be aware of whether any of the more challenging aspects are starting to develop and take steps to counter their development by using the appropriate Bush Essences.

In my first book, *Australian Bush Flower Essences*, I discussed the individual numbers on the grid in great detail. In this book I will focus on one aspect only, known as 'The Arrows'.

The first step in this system of numerology is to write down your child's birth date. Each number in the birth date always has its own spot on the grid, which looks like this:

3	6	9	Mental Plane
2	5	8	Emotional Plane
1	4	7	Physical Plane

The tenth numeral, zero, does not have a place on the grid, but rather represents spiritual potential.

3	6	
2		
1	4	

For example, if you were working with the birth date 16 March 2004, you would express this as 16.3.2004. Then each of the numerals would be written down in its specific place on the grid:

Each place on the grid represents a specific character trait, or aspect of personality. If three numbers appear in a straight line, it is known as an Arrow and is indicative of an inherent strength greater than the sum of the individual three numbers by themselves. The arrows, in fact, reveal either significant strengths or weaknesses. Arrows can run horizontally, vertically or diagonally across the grid.

Most charts have at least one arrow, or three numbers in a straight line. An arrow can also refer to the lack of all three numbers in a row. Young children born so far this millennium will have many missing numbers, so they are likely to have more missing arrows than full arrows.

In all there are sixteen arrows, and in the following pages I will focus on each of them and suggest which Bush Essences would be appropriate for a child having a particular arrow. Of course, the qualities and the recommendations for the specific Bush Essences would be equally applicable for a teenager or an adult with this same arrow.

ARROW OF DETERMINATION

This is the most common arrow among people born in the twentieth century, as everyone from this century has already had the 1 and the 9 and only require the 5 to complete the arrow. Children with this arrow are often very persistent, and if they are also lacking a 4 in their chart they are likely to be highly impatient if their plans are not met as quickly as they would like. They would be more prone to tantrums, have a quick temper and get very frustrated if they are not able to do things, especially if there are older siblings who can do these things. For frustration at not being able to run more quickly or keep up with the others, Wild Potato Bush is the remedy. Black-eyed Susan, which is in Calm and Clear Essence, is the perfect essence for addressing impatience. This essence, by allowing a child to be still and listen to their intuition, can help them realise that if things are not working out as quickly as they want or if obstacles are impeding their plans then it might not be the right timing or the appropriate direction they are following.

If your child has only a single 1, 5 and 9 then the main focus is on the 9, which means she will tend to be idealistic. This is also the case if she has more than one 9 in her birth date. These children become particularly upset if animals, people or the environment are hurt at all. A tendency towards being too idealistic is addressed by the remedy Sundew, which is in Emergency Essence.

If your child has more than one 5 in the grid, she would tend towards emotional intensity. The remedy Crowea would be helpful because, when she is stressed, she is likely to suffer stomach pain. Crowea helps the discomfort around the abdominal area.

ARROW OF PROCRASTINATION

This arrow occurs where there is no 1, 5 or 9 in the birth date. A child with this arrow will have a tendency to put off tasks and activities, or not to start them at all. The Bush Essence Sundew is a wonderful tool to correct this pattern, and the earlier you can work with this essence on a child with the Arrow of Procrastination the better. If either parent has had a tendency to procrastinate then add Boab, or Confid Essence which contains it, for the hereditary component.

Your role as a parent is crucial in helping your child with this arrow. As well as focusing on helping her to initiate and commence tasks, it would be extremely beneficial to either observe or help your child finish that particular activity so that she can develop the habit, and the subsequent satisfaction, of completion.

Other essences to consider when working with the Arrow of Procrastination are: Paw Paw, for feeling too overwhelmed to start; Jacaranda, for being easily side-tracked and not completing tasks and projects; and Peach-flowered Tea-tree, for getting bored and not finishing. All of these are likely to be used along with Sundew. Kapok Bush could also be considered to help develop your child's sense of persistence and not to give up, while Black-eyed Susan would help engender the virtue of patience.

ARROW OF SPIRITUALITY

This arrow is formed when a child has the numbers 3, 5 and 7 in his birth date. Children with this arrow love to be of help to others, especially animals, other children and those in need. The Dalai Lama is a classic example of this. It has been said of him that 'his presence brings peace to all around him'. The 7 in their chart usually means that they prefer to experience life directly in a practical way rather than theoretically. They won't be so interested in advice from others.

The remedy Southern Cross, in Confid Essence, is very useful to children with this arrow because they often have a deep sense of natural justice and can become upset if they feel things 'are not fair' when someone is treated unjustly. The remedy can be used for a child who tends to feel self-pity and blame others for what happens to them.

Many people with the Arrow of Spirituality also display a strong respect for Nature and all forms of life. If your child has this arrow but is not displaying this quality, he could benefit from a dose of Red Helmet Orchid as it is very specific for this aspect.

You may also consider Angelsword for these children to help develop within them a greater sense of discernment as they frequently trust others naively. Meditation Essence, which contains this remedy, can be used to further enhance their interest in spirituality, religion or philosophy, which they are likely to be drawn to.

ARROW OF THE ENQUIRER

This arrow occurs when a child does **not** have the numbers 3, 5 or 7 in her birth date. My numerology teacher, David Phillips, originally referred to it as the Arrow of the Sceptic before adopting the more politically correct name of Arrow of the Enquirer. Both names are very apt. A child with this arrow will generally never accept anything on trust but will want to investigate it for themselves. If she is convinced of the truth of something, she can often become an ardent supporter and defender of it. If, on the other hand, she is not convinced, she is highly unlikely to ever revisit that subject. You could consider Freshwater Mangrove for a child who makes up her mind about something before experiencing it.

Scepticism can be helpful, and many scientists have this arrow. It leads them towards investigation and the seeking of answers. Some people with this arrow can worry about life's uncertainties and their inability to explain life's mysteries. Crowea is the essence for this. Children and teenagers with this arrow can be seen as moody and Peach-flowered Tea-tree will help here, while Turkey Bush will enhance their artistic expression in painting, music or writing, which will soften this arrow and help round out their personalities.

ARROW OF THE INTELLECT

This arrow occurs when a child has the birth date numbers 3, 6 and 9 in what is called the mental plane. A child with this arrow is likely to have an extremely active and well-balanced mind, with a very good memory.

This arrow, when positively expressed, leads to a personality that is inquisitive, bright and happy. Because of their quick grasp of ideas and mental dexterity, children with this arrow often carry a great deal of responsibility both in the home and at school, often becoming class captains, for example. One of their biggest challenges is not to become impatient or overly critical of those around them who are not as quick or mentally gifted as they are. If they have problems dealing with these two issues then both Black-eyed Susan and Yellow Cowslip Orchid respectively can help them.

Because their mind is usually so dominant and they frequently have fewer numbers on the emotional plane, children with this arrow may find it difficult to access their feelings. Bluebell and Flannel Flower will help such an aspect. Fortunately, children born from the year 2000 onwards will all have the number 2 in their birth date, and this enhances intuition and sensitivity.

ARROW OF POOR MEMORY

This is an arrow that will occur commonly in the new millennium. It occurs when a child has no 3, 6 or 9 in their birth date.

In the past, people with this arrow were advised to work conscientiously towards a good memory, with ongoing study and work that required a lot of thinking. However, this current generation of young children are operating far more from their feeling centre, with an innate heightened intuition and sensitivity. This is particularly evident in children being born this millennium who have at least one 2 in their birth chart. The quality for 2 is intuition, sense and sensitivity. I feel that this generation of young children will use their right brain or intuitive, creative side to a much higher degree than previous generations. There will also be more emphasis on knowing and feeling what is appropriate rather than relying on rational, logical thought—not that the latter will not also be necessary.

However, these children will enhance their concentration levels by working with Cognis Essence. It contains Jacaranda, for focus; Bush Fuchsia, for integrating the two hemispheres of the brain; and Sundew, for attention to detail. Isopogon, the Bush Essence specific for memory and recall, would be an important remedy for anyone with this arrow.

I think there is great merit today in Rudolf Steiner's educational model and philosophy for children. He advocates a later starting time for certain academic subjects such as mathematics, placing a greater emphasis on soul development and connection to Nature when children are younger. It is likely that children having the Arrow of Poor Memory will be more open and responsive to thought and ideas compared to more traditional left-brain focused generations.

ARROW OF EMOTIONAL BALANCE

You find this arrow in a birth date with 2, 5 and 8, the numbers on the emotional plane, all present. This will be one of the most common arrows in charts until the year 3000.

A child with the Arrow of Emotional Balance is likely to be both very sensitive and intuitive. Usually these children enjoy helping others, and as they get older are quite likely to work professionally as counsellors or healers as they have a natural ability to read and understand others.

Children with this arrow can become quite serious and even withdrawn. Regular doses of Little Flannel Flower will be of great benefit, helping them to be more light-hearted and carefree. They make very good actors as they have the capacity for excellent emotional control. They are able to harness the sensitivity and perceptions of others to bring alive and make very real and believable the characters they are portraying.

Generally, these children strongly identify and pick up on emotional conflicts happening around them and especially so if they are directly involved. Frequently their response will be to withdraw as a mechanism to avoid such conflict. Tall Mulla Mulla is an excellent essence to use if you observe this trait developing in a child with this arrow. If they have more than one 2 in their birth date they may tend to take on the emotions of others around them, and Fringed Violet will help with this. Obviously, the avoidance of very violent, noisy or excessively melodramatic movies or TV would be recommended for these children as they are overly impressionable and can be easily affected by such programs.

ARROW OF HYPERSENSITIVITY

3	6	9
←		
11		7

This arrow occurs when 2, 5 and 8, the numbers on the emotional plane, are all missing from the birth date.

Children with this arrow are likely to be very shy and sensitive, and also quite timid and anxious. They may have difficulty relating to their peers, and can be loners. Usually their self-esteem and confidence will be low. Confid Essence can bring about startling transformations in these young beings, helping them to develop a great deal of confidence and courage and giving a big boost to their self-esteem.

These children usually crave a lot of love and have a tendency to be quite clingy. If a young child, especially a boy (as they generally suffer greater separation anxiety than young girls), with this arrow was placed regularly in childcare when under the age of four, and especially under the age of three, he is likely to experience a great deal more emotional trauma and upset than other children. Ideally, such placements should be kept to a minimum. If parents do decide on more daycare for such children, then these essences would be of great value to the child: Bottlebrush for both bonding to the mother and letting go; Illawarra Flame Tree for feelings of rejection; and Tall Yellow Top for feelings of abandonment.

Because they are easily hurt, these children often develop as a defence mechanism a tough exterior or external persona which they use to hide their true sensitive, gentle nature. Alternatively, some can develop a very harsh or prickly persona designed to stop people getting close to them, for they feel that if someone does get close that either they will hurt them or they will end up hurt. Pink Mulla Mulla is a wonderful essence for these patterns and helps to disarm the prickles and armouring that has been built up for protection.

ARROW OF PRACTICALITY

The Arrow of Practicality contains the numbers 1, 4 and 7, which are all on the physical plane. These are the 'doing' people of the world. Some children with this arrow have been misdiagnosed as hyperactive because they have so much energy and they never seem to stop—but it's just that they have loads of stamina.

Commonly, these children are very skilful in working with their hands. If they are not utilising this potential then either Flannel Flower, to help them enjoy expressing themselves physically, or Five Corners, to develop their confidence in trusting their manual capabilities, should correct the situation.

A challenge that may arise for children with this arrow as they mature is a tendency to be overly materialistic and strongly motivated by worldly desires and materialistic ambition. Bush Iris is very effective in addressing this trait, while Pink Flannel Flower would help them learn gratitude and Bluebell would help them with generosity and sharing.

These people are, on a deeper level, usually very sensitive, though others may not appreciate this aspect and be misled by their more robust, practical and active approach to life. Interestingly enough, I have observed that many with the Arrow of Practicality have an affinity to music. Either they have a great appreciation of it or music is exceptionally healing for them. The music on the White Light CD in particular can have a tremendously deep impact on them, as would being in direct contact with Nature.

I have also noticed a degree of stubbornness with many of these children, and Isopogon would be indicated if this is the case.

ARROW OF DISORDER

When the numbers 1, 4 and 7 are all missing from the birth date, you have the Arrow of Disorder. It is very common for children who have been born in the new millennium to have no numbers on the physical plane.

The greatest challenge these children will face is in leading focused, orderly lives. It is likely that they will also have to battle the tendency of being overly theoretical or idealistic and not completing projects. Jacaranda will address a tendency towards dithering or being scattered, with their attention being taken to a new area before they have finished the task that they are currently on.

Black-eyed Susan will help these children learn patience and might be an especially useful remedy for their parents and educators, who will be attempting to teach them this very same thing. I would suggest that great benefit would occur if these children could be taught, in a practical way, the satisfaction of finishing simple tasks and of not starting new projects until the old one is finished. Jacaranda is excellent for this. I would even suggest financial reward could be considered upon the completion of such tasks and projects to facilitate them learning this important lesson.

Working in the garden would also help these children, allowing them to understand the intricacies of Nature and to see the rewards that can be reaped from work. It should not be too hard to entice these children into the garden as they are likely to have a natural inclination to embracing conservation and ecology. There is a high likelihood that with this arrow they will be untidy as well, and Hibbertia can help instil a degree of internal order and discipline for them.

Having no numbers on the physical plane, the thoughts and ideas of these children are likely to be centred on the external world and not so much on themselves. They are likely to be idealistic and willing to put self secondary to the common good, and they have the potential to be very motivated to support and assist organisations and projects they strongly believe in.

You could consider Flannel Flower if your child has this arrow. It will support him in expressing himself physically, as there may be a tendency for him to have a sedentary lifestyle focusing on computers, PlayStations and so on rather than running around and being active in his play.

ARROW OF THE PLANNER

The Arrow of the Planner joins the first numbers on each of the three planes and will be the most commonly found arrow in the 21st century. This line indicates creative imagination, together with thoughts and plans concerning others and the community at large. Individuals with this arrow will usually be able to receive or develop many inspired plans. It will be especially interesting to observe in this century as many children with this arrow are also likely to have more than one 2 in their birth chart. This will accentuate their intuitive abilities so that they can be more readily inspired and conceive ideas through both their guides and spirit.

When Arrow of the Planner people are under pressure or in a crisis they can be so caught up in their own thoughts and plans they can be unaware of the needs of others. Kangaroo Paw is the perfect essence for this and Calm and Clear Essence will also be good. The latter will prevent them from getting in that state in the first place. They are very good problem solvers and trouble shooters for others and love helping people find a solution, even when the issue is complex.

Children with the Arrow of the Planner will derive great pleasure from organising plans, even if quite small, for themselves, friends or family, so do encourage them in this area. One can often observe a nervous restlessness with children having this arrow, due to them being so much in their mind, being so absorbed in their thoughts and plans, that they are often unaware of how to manifest them or how to convert their mental energy into physical activity. Flannel Flower will help these children to express themselves physically. Ironically, even though anyone with this arrow will often have a need and desire for ordered method, there can be a tendency for these people to neglect practical details. They tend to be more concerned with the big picture and the function of organising rather than putting the plan into action; if so, Sundew will help them.

THE ARROW OF WILL

The Arrow of Will occurs when your child has 4, 5 and 6 in her birth date. Anyone with this arrow has a great drive to succeed, together with a very strong willpower to help them achieve this ambition.

Some of the power and drive associated with this arrow can be explained by the fact that it contains the central point of the mental, emotional and physical planes. When in balance, so much can be achieved: both Leonardo Da Vinci and Shakespeare had this arrow in their birth chart. However, one of the greatest challenges is that these people have so much drive and energy that they overpower those around them. In many cases this can preclude a person with this arrow from achieving greatness.

As well, children with this arrow often fail to take advice from others as they are so clearly focused on and set in pursuing their own course. They may have clashes of will with their parents, teachers or siblings. Gymea Lily is a very beneficial remedy for them, enabling them to take a back seat rather than always being the leader. Others around them will benefit from gaining the opportunity to contribute more to leadership, especially younger brothers or sisters.

Bush Fuchsia will greatly help someone with this arrow to develop their intuition. If they can slow down long enough to listen and follow their intuition, they can then put their energy and drive to work in the right direction. Black-eyed Susan would help them because Arrow of the Will people can often become very irritated and annoyed by people who are not as energised, focused, quick and driven as they themselves are. Both these remedies are found in Calm and Clear Essence.

These children often have a sense of direction, though even without one they will charge forward and are likely to create one along the way. Calm and Clear Essence drops or cream can be very beneficial for these children, especially at night to help them slow down, unwind and have a good night's sleep.

ARROW OF FRUSTRATION

This is one of the most common arrows that you will find in the chart of people born since 1970. People with this arrow are missing 4, 5 and 6, the centre numbers from all three planes, in the chart—the mental, emotional and physical.

With the Arrow of Frustration there can often seem to be a lack of both willpower and tenacity and a personality with the tendency to give up quite easily. Kapok Bush would be the essence indicated for this trait. Children with this arrow will benefit from developing the strength and resilience to overcome the various challenges they are likely to encounter. Unfortunately they usually experience a lot more challenges than most people, and especially so in their own eyes. In my numerology workshops I mention that a common phrase people with this arrow regularly utter, especially those younger ones, is 'It's not fair!', and many a participant has a wry laugh. These are usually the parents of such children. The remedy for this arrow is Southern Cross, which brilliantly matches the victim mentality that you frequently find associated with this arrow. It is for that sense of 'Why me?' Southern Cross will assist a child to realise that life isn't something that just happens to them but rather that they can help shape and create the reality they want through their thoughts, intentions, beliefs and actions.

At the same time, this essence can stop them being despondent and left with a chip on their shoulder. Southern Cross will help them become aware of the silver lining of every cloud and to realise that nothing happens by accident. It is not uncommon for children with this arrow to have parents who are separating, as well as difficulties and challenges with money, health and relationships in their life. Pink Flannel Flower assists children to see all the wonderful things in their lives and focus on these rather than the occasional disappointment or challenge, and it will help restore their joie de vivre.

As they mature, the remedy Monga Waratah will help them to learn the very important lesson of standing on their own two feet and being independent. If you see this trait in a child with this arrow, the earlier you can start using this essence the better.

THE ARROW OF ACTIVITY

When I first started studying numerology, anyone having the numbers 7, 8 and 9 present in their birth date was said to have the Arrow of Hyperactivity. It was emphasised that anyone having this arrow, especially children and teenagers, would be very prone to allergies as well as having strong reactions to any artificial colours and preservatives in their diet. All of this could commonly lead to learning and behavioural problems (see 'Food intolerance' on page 153). Fringed Violet decreases any reactivity that they may have to pollutants as well as chemicals in both the environment and in the food they ingest.

A person with what is now called the Arrow of Activity has a great deal of nervous energy. Many with this arrow are easily distracted and scattered in their energy, are highly strung and tend to be a little flighty. Jacaranda is indicated for all these traits. Children with this arrow growing up in, or having access to, the country with plenty of greenery and wide open space around them usually fare a whole lot better than their peers growing in an urban environment, especially in high-rise apartment buildings, with little open space around them. Crowea is a wonderful remedy to help bring balance to a child with this aspect in their chart.

The Creative Essence combination would also be highly beneficial to a child with this arrow as it helps with emotional expression, allowing and encouraging him to express a dramatic flair and innate creativity. It's when individuals with this arrow aren't able to express themselves that problems develop. In adolescent years these can manifest in increased rebellious behaviour, and Red Helmet Orchid can help here.

THE ARROW OF PASSIVITY

3		↑
2	5	
	4	

This arrow, where the numbers 7, 8 and 9 are all missing from the birth date, started to occur in the year 2000, after a long absence dating back to December 1666. Any child born with the Arrow of Passivity will benefit greatly from regular doses of Kapok Bush. There will be a tendency for these children not to have the necessary drive to physically follow through and achieve what they wish to accomplish.

Essences to consider for children with the Arrow of Passivity include both Sundew, to keep them grounded, and Flannel Flower, to help them physically express themselves. Dynamis Combination, too, could be used for extra stamina and energy.

Their biggest challenge may be simply getting around to commencing tasks, and Kapok Bush addresses this. Hibbertia will also help instil a sense of discipline to include physical activity and exercise at home and at school. One of the important benefits of anyone having this arrow is their inclination to live a peaceful and harmonious life.

This is in sharp contrast to the numbers 1 and 9, which are present in everyone's birth date from the twentieth century—the bloodiest century in human history, where over one hundred million people were killed in violent conflicts and war. I see Pink Flannel Flower as a marvellous remedy to accentuate the awareness and appreciation of all the wonderful things present in life and of this planet that a child with this arrow is likely to feel.

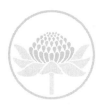

12

CHOOSING BUSH ESSENCES

I've found that when people first learn about the properties of Bush Essences, they often say they need to take many of the remedies instantly. That's how strongly they identify with them. This common response shows the beautiful simplicity of the essences. And it isn't just yourself that you see in the remedies, but also all the people you know and love. You don't need years of formal training to have this instant insight, but just a basic understanding of human nature.

Throughout this book I have suggested appropriate remedies for particular conditions or issues. If you are new to Bush Essences, my suggestions will guide you in your choice of remedies so that even when you or your child needs help for a very specific situation, you can choose the appropriate essence.

It is usually quite easy to choose essences for children because what they are feeling tends to be obvious. You don't need medical or psychological training to see when a child is suffering from a lack of confidence, or is feeling insecure or sad.

Sometimes you may need to observe more closely. What change is your child going through? Has something happened recently to upset him? Listen for clues when your child is talking to you or interacting with others. Are there things going on in the family that might unsettle her, even though you aren't speaking openly about what's happening? Keep in mind that children quickly pick up on what's happening around them.

Once you have an idea of how your child is feeling, either read through the descriptions of the individual essences and select the one that's most relevant, or refer to the repertory to find the remedies that match her condition.

You can also use the Flower Insight Cards or the photos of the flowers in the colour section of this book. Simply lay the cards out on a table or on the floor or turn to the colour section and ask your child to choose the three flowers they like best. You can then talk about the qualities of these flowers as described in Chapter 15 and ask her if she can relate to any of these aspects. Or else shuffle the cards and ask her to randomly choose one without looking at the images. You can trust that she will choose the flowers whose essences will be most beneficial to her.

COMBINATION ESSENCES

Many Bush Essences are included in combination essences such as Emergency Essence or Calm and Clear Essence. If a particular essence is suggested, you can give your child that individual essence or you can give a combination essence that contains it.

For example, Emergency Essence drops contains:

- Angelsword;
- Crowea;
- Dog Rose of the Wild Forces;
- Fringed Violet;
- Grey Spider Flower;
- Sundew; and
- Waratah.

If Crowea is suggested for a condition, Emergency Essence will provide you with it, along with the benefits of the other essences included in the combination. If any of the essences contained in the combination essence drops, mists and creams are not needed they simply will not have any effect.

I've taken this approach throughout the book. This way, by utilising combination essences, you have a good number of Bush Essences at hand. Combination essences are readily available from my company, Australian Bush Flower Essences, directly, or at health food stores, selected pharmacies and from many natural health practitioners.

INDIVIDUAL ESSENCES AND THE COMBINATION ESSENCE IN WHICH THEY CAN BE FOUND

Alpine Mint Bush (not contained in a combination)

Angelsword (Emergency, Meditation, Space Clearing)

Autumn Leaves (Transition)

Banksia Robur (Dynamis, Travel)

Bauhinia (Purifying, Transition)

Billy Goat Plum (Adol, Face, Hand and Body cream, Sensuality, Sexuality, Woman)

Black-eyed Susan (Calm and Clear)

Bluebell (Abund, Relationship)

Boab (Abund, Adol, Confid, Relationship, Space Clearing)

Boronia (Calm and Clear, Meditation)

Bottlebrush (Adol, Calm and Clear, Purifying, Relationship, Transition, Travel, Woman)

Bush Fuchsia (Calm and Clear, Cognis, Creative, Electro, Meditation, Travel, Woman)

Bush Gardenia (Relationship, Sensuality, Sexuality)

Bush Iris (Meditation, Purifying, Transition, Travel)

Christmas Bell (Abund)

Crowea (Emergency, Calm and Clear, Creative, Dynamis, Electro, Travel, Woman)

Dagger Hakea (Adol, Purifying, Relationship)

Dog Rose (Confid, Purifying)

Dog Rose of the Wild Forces (Emergency)

Five Corners (Abund, Adol, Confid, Creative, Face, Hand and Body cream, Woman)

Flannel Flower (Adol, Creative, Face, Hand and Body cream, Relationship, Sensuality Mist, Sexuality)

Freshwater Mangrove (not contained in a combination)

Fringed Violet (Electro, Emergency, Meditation, Sexuality, Space Clearing, Travel)

Green Essence (not contained in a combination)

Green Spider Orchid (Meditation)

Grey Spider Flower (Emergency)

Gymea Lily (not contained in a combination)

Hibbertia (not contained in a combination)

Illawarra Flame Tree (Dynamis)

Isopogon (Cognis)

Jacaranda (Calm and Clear, Cognis)

Kangaroo Paw (Adol)

Kapok Bush (not contained in a combination)

Lichen (Space Clearing, Transition)

Little Flannel Flower (Calm and Clear, Face, Hand and Body cream, Sensuality, Sexuality)

Macrocarpa (Dynamis, Sensuality, Travel)

Mint Bush (Relationship, Transition)

Monga Waratah (not contained in a combination)

Mountain Devil (not contained in a combination)

Mulla Mulla (Electro, Face, Hand and Body cream, Solaris, Travel, Woman)

Old Man Banksia (Dynamis, Woman)

Paw Paw (Calm and Clear, Cognis, Electro, Travel)

Peach-flowered Tea-tree (Woman)

Philotheca (Abund)

Pink Flannel Flower (Abund, Woman)

Pink Mulla Mulla (not contained in a combination)

Red Grevillea (Creative, Transition)

Red Helmet Orchid (Adol, Relationship)

Red Lily (Meditation, Space Clearing, Travel)

Red Suva Frangipani (Relationship)

Rough Bluebell (not contained in a combination)

She Oak (Face, Hand and Body cream, Solaris, Travel, Woman)

Silver Princess (Transition, Travel)

Slender Rice Flower (Emergency Essence cream only, not the drops or mist)

Southern Cross (Abund, Adol, Confid)

Spinifex (Emergency cream only, not the drops or mist, Solaris)

CHOOSING BUSH ESSENCES

Sturt Desert Pea (not contained in a combination)
Sturt Desert Rose (Confid, Sensuality, Sexuality)
Sundew (Emergency, Cognis, Travel)
Sunshine Wattle (Abund, Adol)
Sydney Rose (not contained in a combination)
Tall Mulla Mulla (Creative, Travel)
Tall Yellow Top (Adol)
Turkey Bush (Creative)
Yellow Cowslip Orchid (Dynamis)
Waratah (Electro, Emergency)
Wedding Bush (Relationship)
Wild Potato Bush (Purifying)
Wisteria (Face, Hand and Body cream, Sensuality, Sexuality)
Yellow Cowslip Orchid (Dynamis)

You will find a detailed list of the essences and the issues they address in Chapter 15.

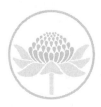

13

USING BUSH ESSENCES

The standard Bush Essence dose is 7 drops from the dosage bottle, under the tongue, first thing in the morning and last thing at night. These times of the day are powerful periods for the psyche, and at the same time they make it very easy for you to remember to take them or give them to your child.

If the remedy is for an emotional imbalance you would usually take it or give it to your child for two weeks, but if you are addressing a physical problem it would usually need to be taken for at least a month. There is no harm in taking the remedy for longer periods.

If the alcohol in a remedy is a problem for children, you can add the drops to a glass of hot water and allow the alcohol to evaporate. Your child can then drink the glass of water once it has cooled. A remedy can also be applied topically. Simply rub it onto the wrists or forehead, or onto the sore limb or sore stomach.

Some of the combination essences are also available as mists, such as Emergency Essence which has a calming effect during a crisis. Space Clearing Essence is a mist which purifies and releases the environment of built-up negative energies. Calm and Clear can be sprayed in your child's bedroom before she goes to bed to help her settle down quickly.

A lesson in essences

Shelley Sishton, a practitioner from the United Kingdom who uses the essences avidly and with great results, could never convince her client, a kindergarten teacher, to use the remedies. One day the teacher complained how noisy the children were and how stressed she was and that she had started to yell at the class. Shelley offered her Emergency Essence spray saying, 'Just spray it around the classroom.' The teacher was so at her wit's end she decided she had nothing to lose even though she knew it wouldn't work. To her great surprise, she was amazed how quickly after she sprayed the room the children calmed down, stopped talking, paid attention and were able to follow her instructions. After a few days of spraying, another kindergarten teacher came into her classroom at lunchtime and asked what was happening as she had noticed such a huge difference in the first teacher's class. Shelley's client replied, 'Well, I tried this spray. I don't know if it is that which is doing it or not.' The other teacher asked if she could try some and she too had similar excellent results. A week later the headmistress called Shelley's client into her office to find out what was going on in the two classrooms, as the whole school had noticed the huge difference. The teacher explained how she had been using Emergency Essence spray, saying, 'Well, I'm not sure if it's coincidence but things seem to be happening with it.' The headmistress sheepishly asked if her room could be sprayed because she had a difficult meeting with some very aggressive parents that afternoon. The next morning the headmistress bailed up Shelley's client to tell her that something amazing had happened: for the first time in fifteen years she'd had a really good night's sleep and the meeting had gone really well, and she wanted to know if her room could be sprayed again and if she could get a second good night's sleep. The next day the headmistress complained to her, 'It couldn't have been the Emergency Essence because last night I didn't have a good sleep at all.' The teacher then confessed that she had been so busy she hadn't had time to spray the headmistress's room yesterday but went and got the spray and did it then. The next day the headmistress reported another good night's sleep. The whole school is currently using Emergency Essence spray!

Ian

FIRST AID

Accidents

Whatever the accident, a child is less likely to panic if the people around him are calm and focused, so it is important that you are able to be as serene as possible when your child is distressed. Emergency Essence comes into its own with any kind of accident. It takes a way a lot of the pain, shock, stress and trauma involved, both for your child and for you, too.

I recommend that every household has a bottle of Emergency Essence because a high number of accidents occur in the home. Also keep a bottle in the car; you never know when you may come across a traffic accident or an injured animal. The essence comes in cream form as well as a spray, but you are most likely to use it in drop form. It is a wonderful remedy for day-to-day accidents and upsets. Sometimes children get quite a shock at having a fall, and Emergency Essence will calm them very quickly. You'll find that within 30 seconds, a child who has fallen off a bike or tripped over has stopped crying and is running around having forgotten all about the accident. The essence can be used every ten minutes or so, then tapered off as the pain lessens. Emergency Essence cream can be applied to bruises, swellings, strains and sprains.

Sports injuries

A marathon runner was training on a Thursday when he crashed into a gate and badly bruised his knee, which swelled up very quickly. As he hobbled back to his car his running partner said, 'Oh, there goes your marathon this Saturday.' His wife had done a Bush Essence workshop a few months earlier but had never been able to convince him Bush Essences were effective. When he got home he thought he'd give these flower essences a try to see if they really did work. He smothered his knee in Emergency Essence cream, and then again before going to bed. The next morning he woke up and the swelling had dropped remarkably, and he continued using Emergency Essence drops and cream the next day and was able to run his marathon. As he told me at the next workshop he came to: 'I was a real sceptic but I know enough about my body and running to know that there was no

way I could have competed in that marathon without Emergency Essence. This stuff really works!'
Ian

Emergency Essence is also great for other sports injuries, whether it's being pushed over at netball, falling off a horse or being bruised in a contact sport. One of the remedies in this essence, Crowea, works on the muscles and tendons and so addresses any strains and sprains. The Fringed Violet in Emergency Essence will release emotional and physical shock. This is important, because if shock is not released from the body after an accident it remains in your child's body at a cellular level, where it can cause damage. Fringed Violet has the ability to go back in time, years earlier if necessary, to the original incident to release any traumas held in the body. It's a good essence for parents to consider for themselves, too.

Bites and stings

Some children are very curious about insects and will pick them up to inspect them. If they are bitten or stung, Emergency Essence will ease any pain and swelling. It is a great remedy for any bites and stings. Always take it with you on holidays, or for trips down to the beach or when you are camping in the bush.

At the beach, it is not unusual for bluebottles to be around. These days the recommended treatment is an application of hot water, usually a hot shower. The hot water will neutralise the sting. Taking Emergency Essence frequently will help to deal with the pain, and it will also help with any allergic reactions or swelling of the lymph glands.

If your child suffers from mosquito bites, midges or ticks apply Emergency Essence cream or drops to the bites to reduce any irritation and swelling and to ease the itching.

Spiders and snakes
In the case of either a spider or snake bite, use a bandage to apply pressure to the bite and make sure your child remains still. Any movement can help spread the flow of the toxin

and is highly dangerous, so it is essential that the child is still while someone gets medical help. Emergency Essence drops will help to calm your child until help arrives.

When you are going out into the bush, always pack a number of bandages together with Emergency Essence in case such an event happens.

Broken bones

If your child suffers a broken bone in an accident, Emergency Essence will address the initial pain, shock and trauma. There are two further remedies that will actually help heal the bones: the first is Gymea Lily, which works on ligaments and bones, and the other is Hibbertia, which stimulates the parathyroid, involved in the production of calcium, and so helps speed up the healing of the broken bone. These two remedies can be added to Emergency Essence and taken for two or three weeks after the accident. After that, the two remedies can be given without Emergency Essence.

Bruises

When a bruise first occurs you can use Emergency drops internally or the cream topically to help reduce pain and any shock. If the blood vessels have broken very easily it can be a sign of vitamin C deficiency. Tall Mulla Mulla strenghtens the blood vessels and I would give this as well. For children who are constantly bruising themselves you might consider Bush Fuchsia so they will become more coordinated and not as likely to have so many accidents, and Black-eyed Susan to help slow them down from being like a bull in a china shop. Both essences are in Calm and Clear Essence. Children not getting enough sleep may also be more accident prone and again Calm and Clear Essence can help them get good quality sleep at night.

Burns

Children can easily suffer minor burns around the home. The Solaris combination, which contains Mulla Mulla, is a great first aid remedy in case your child puts a hand on the heater, gets scalded in the bath, pulls something off the stove, or suffers sunburn. In the case of such a burn, you can give your child Solaris or the remedy Mulla Mulla every ten or fifteen minutes.

Healing burns

I have been amazed at the instant effects [of the essences] on burns. Cameron only believes that something is hot by touching it, and therefore we have had hot water burns a lot, not serious but enough to raise redness in the skin and a great deal of discomfort for him. With a few drops of Mulla Mulla on the area the redness disappears in minutes and the sting even quicker. When my children burn their mouths on hot food, a few drops in the mouth and there is no evidence of any tenderness or blistering. In fact, when Michael now burns his mouth he doesn't even bother to tell me, he just yells, 'Get the drops, quick!'

Janne Ferguson, Victoria, Australia

Solaris is very effective even with third-degree burns. There are numerous case histories where people (including children with third-degree burns) have taken Mulla Mulla drops every half hour and the healing has been so complete they have not needed skin grafts. Children will stay calm, and the essence also eases the pain and the trauma. Once you destroy the top layer of the skin it is very easy for infections to occur, but by using Mulla Mulla the healing happens so quickly, it rarely does.

Burnt skin

Casey had a blocked nose and decided to use a steam tent. About five seconds after pouring the just-boiled water into a large bowl, she accidentally pulled the whole bowl off the table and over her stomach. To make matters worse, she was wearing a bikini top with a metal ring.

We placed her into a cool bath—her stomach and legs were red raw—and rang an ambulance. While we waited I put about five squirts of Mulla Mulla under her tongue and put half a bottle of Mulla Mulla stock into the bathwater. By the time the ambulance arrived there was virtually no sign of any burn marks on her skin at all. She was still very sore of course but they couldn't believe that her skin wasn't totally blistered. I then gave her She Oak in water to hydrate the skin and today there are no visible signs of burns at all.

Julie Tucker, address withheld on request

If your child is burnt, run the area under cool water for up to twenty or 30 minutes, giving Mulla Mulla frequently. Burns to the face are very dangerous and medical assistance is required urgently, but keep giving Mulla Mulla drops to relieve the pain and to help quick recovery.

Severe burns

Taylah poured boiling water from microwave-cooked food down her arm, scalding it terribly. She was hospitalised with deep blistering burns from her fingers to her elbow. I prescribed orally Dagger Hakea, Mountain Devil and Mulla Mulla.

Her dressing had to stay on for about three weeks and then she would need a possible skin graft. When her dressing was taken off her hand to the wrist, she had open blisters on her fingers and the back of the hand. I made a spray with Spinifex, Bush Iris, Slender Rice Flower, Mulla Mulla and She Oak. In three days her hand had dried and peeled and there were two small pink marks on her hand. When her dressing came off, I immediately began using the spray on her arm. At this stage the doctors still had concerns that Taylah would need a skin graft. They had decided to give the arm one more week to see how it healed.

In the first 24 hours of using the spray Taylah's arm healed more than in the three weeks prior. In three days the burn had 'lifted' and sealed and Taylah had dead skin dropping off rapidly. I say 'lifted' because the burn seemed to come to the surface rather than remain deep in the tissue of her arm. I prescribed Bush Iris and Slender Rice Flower to help prevent scarring,

Mulla Mulla for the burn, Spinifex to stop infection and She Oak to rehydrate tissue. No skin graft! Go Flower Power!

Tahli Tremayne, Victoria, Australia

Mulla Mulla is also a very good remedy even many years after a bad burn. It releases the trauma from the body, and also helps with healing the scarring from the burn. This remedy is also good for those children who don't like the heat and are affected by hot days during the summer months.

Stinging eyes

My daughter, aged seven, was playing outside, making a 'magic potion' with herbs and items from the garden. She opened a chilli she found, scraped out the seeds, and rubbed her eye. Next thing, she was screaming and crying 'My eye, my eye'. Initially she started washing her eye with water which didn't help. Knowing the cause I gave her Mulla Mulla and within seconds she had calmed down and there was less stinging. Five minutes later I gave her more Mulla Mulla and the redness around her face from the rubbing had eased. She went back outside to play.

Jane Borgeaud, Australian Captial Territory

Cuts

Where cuts are more superficial and not requiring stitches, give Emergency Essence for the shock, and the remedy Spinifex to help heal fine cuts. If it is a deeper cut requiring stitching, then give the remedy Slender Rice Flower. Such deep cuts invariably affect any meridian that the cut dissects. Slender Rice Flower will restore the energy flow of the meridians when they have been crossed by a cut. Sometimes I have patients in their sixties who have had scars from childhood, and since that time the meridian has not flowed effectively. It is very important to get in early so that children don't have this experience.

Always wash the cut under tap water, and then apply a bandage firmly to stop the flow of blood. Give Emergency Essence every fifteen minutes or so. If it's a very serious cut and the artery has been severed, there will be a lot of spurting blood. Apply a bandage with firm pressure, but be careful not to cut off the blood supply. Then immediately call for an ambulance, keeping your child still until it arrives.

Falls

After a bad fall your child's vertebrae can go out of alignment, affecting nerves that supply his muscles and organs. This may cause the muscles to spasm, and Emergency Essence rubbed into the area will relax the muscles that will allow the vertebrae to go back in place and consequently ease the pain. If your child is having headaches, then give Bush Fuchsia and Boab internally. Both these remedies work on the cranio-sacral areas. Falls can jam up these delicate cranial bones and consequently affect the child's learning capacity if not treated. For any falls affecting the head: monitor the child for four hours; don't let them go to sleep; and if there is any sign of vomiting or if pain is still present after four hours seek medical attention. If there is any continuing pain from a fall the child should also be taken to a health practitioner.

Head injuries

Babies and toddlers have some unique anatomical features that can lead to a higher rate of head injuries. Their heads are larger in proportion to the size of their bodies than adults, and their skull is much less thick than the adult skull. In fact, it is not until about the age of fifteen that the skull is about the same thickness as an adult's.

Children are more prone than adults to suffer bruising of the brain because there is less myelin, a soft, fatty substance, around the nerves. What might be for an adult a painful blow to the head without any long-term damage can be quite traumatic for a child and have a lot of severe physical consequences. Spinifex is a remedy for damaged nerve endings. It is in Emergency Essence cream, but you could also consider adding spinifex to Emergency Essence drops when there has been a head injury.

Also in Emergency Essence is Sundew. If there has been a loss of consciousness, then Sundew will help that. Even for children who have been in comas, Emergency Essence can be applied topically around the temples and on the wrists on a regular basis to help them regain consciousness.

Important: If your child loses consciousness, take him to hospital for a full check-up or medical treatment. The most critical time after any head injury is the first four hours, during which Emergency Essence can be given frequently. Your child should be kept awake during this four-hour period and watched for any signs of vomiting, headaches or loss of coordination. Seek medical help if this occurs.

Recovering from head injuries

One of my ladies said that her son was involved in a car accident and suffered brain damage so severe that he was in a coma for a week. She said that her whole family used Emergency Essence to get them through and misted it through the hospital room. When the son started rehabilitation she started him on Cognis Essence and within weeks there were amazing improvements, the doctors were stunned and she said that the MRI scans showed regeneration of the damaged areas of the brain. I thought that this was an amazing story.

Jasmin Greenough, Western Australia

In the early days of Bush Essences I never mixed them together—I only used them singularly, probably due to my homoeopathic background. Emergency Essence came into being as a result of similar cases to the one above. One of my patients was involved in a very bad car accident witnessed by her husband; she was in a coma in intensive care and was not expected to live. Her husband arrived on my doorstep very distressed, saying he had a sense that I had something I could do to help her. I intuitively mixed a number of remedies together which I gave to him and this was the first time I had ever combined essences. He came back a week later wanting more and said that even when, after three days, his wife came out of the coma the doctors told him not to expect the same person that he had known before the accident because there had been such severe head injuries. However, by the end of that week she was back to her old self again. The doctors were amazed and said they couldn't put it down to anything except the drops she'd been given. Frequently I have received case histories similar to this, with the use of Emergency Essence in particular. In my workshops I always suggest to people to keep a bottle in their car and in their home; you never know when a crisis might arise.

Nosebleeds

Nosebleeds usually indicate that a child needs greater psychic protection. Fringed Violet is a wonderful remedy to address this.

Nosebleeds

Our young son had constant, heavy nosebleeds, particularly at night—once they started they'd continue for a couple of weeks. It greatly upset us all. His doctor suggested that he have his nose cauterised. We were not happy with this idea, so we tried Illawarra Flame Tree instead as I believe his nosebleeds were related to how accepted he's feeling amongst his peers at any given time—his nosebleeds coincide with having a difficult time with his mates. Illawarra Flame Tree stops the nosebleed in a day which are now very rare.

Salvina Syøholm, New South Wales, Australia

Scars

Use Slender Rice Flower to clear any scarring, especially where there are stitches. Give it for two weeks, although sometimes you'll find it clears before that time.

One of the things about scars is that emotions usually get locked into them. Usually when a child has an accident they are out of balance in some way. Perhaps they've had a fight with a sibling; perhaps they're upset and distracted, and so the accident happens. They fall off their bike, for example, or trip over. If they were feeling angry at the time of the accident, this emotion gets locked into the scar. By working with Slender Rice Flower, you release the emotion.

It's the same with surgery: in Chinese medicine, particular emotions are associated with the different organs and parts of the body; fear, for example, affects the kidneys, grief for lungs. Usually there is an emotion triggering the imbalance that leads to the need for surgery. Slender Rice Flower will help to heal the scar and will also release the emotion associated with that organ from the scar.

Skinned knees

Cleanse the skinned area with water to remove any gravel or other foreign material. When it is as clean as possible, the area can be sprayed with Emergency Essence. It may sting a little, but it will really speed up the healing. If you don't have Emergency Essence in spray form, you can apply a few of the oral drops to the skinned area. Also, give your child Emergency Essence drops orally to deal with the pain and any shock.

Sunburn

Children's skin can be easily burnt especially if they are fair haired and fair skinned, so make sure your child always wears protection from the sun. That means wearing a hat that also covers the nape of the neck, if it is exposed, and light, long-sleeved clothes if the sun is fierce. It's best to keep your child out of the sun during the middle hours of the day during the summer.

Children need some sunshine to help make vitamin D in their bodies, which is essential for a healthy immune system and proper bone strength. Giving the child a dose of Mulla Mulla or applying Solaris onto their skin before going out in the sun will help them from absorbing as much of the sun's solar radiation and will lessen skin damage. An extended outdoor summer luncheon picnic can easily result in sun damage for a child of any skin type if they are not protected. Mulla Mulla is in Solaris Essence, which is also a good one to spray onto any sunburn to ease the pain and heal any burning or blistering. It will often stop any peeling. Take orally every fifteen to 30 minutes and apply topically at the same time.

Sunblock

Add 7 drops from the Mulla Mulla stock bottle to every 15 grams of sunblock cream to enhance the sunblock.

Ian

Sunburn

Sarah was very badly sunburnt on Monday. I saw her on Thursday afternoon when her skin was blistered and weeping. I gave her a bottle of Mulla Mulla the next afternoon and directed her to bathe the affected area morning and night and to take the drops internally as well. I also gave her a cream (Sorbolene based) with Mulla Mulla added and told her to apply it after bathing the area.

I saw her again the next Thursday afternoon and was amazed at the condition of her skin. I couldn't even tell where the sunburn had been and there had been no peeling at all. She told me that it had been like that since the previous Sunday— after only one and a half days of using the essence.

Ian

Blisters from sunburn

A little boy was at the beach all day and, although sun cream had been applied, because he is very fair skinned, he came home very burnt. Of particular concern were two burn blisters on each shoulder. I meticulously applied Mulla Mulla on the skin and also gave it to him by mouth every half hour for a few hours. The next morning the blisters had calmed down and the parts of his body that had been red and angry were back to normal. The blisters healed over the next few days and left no scarring or damage to the skin.

J. Cody, New South Wales, Australia

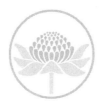

14

A–Z OF CONDITIONS AND TREATMENTS

This A–Z of conditions and treatments contains an alphabetical listing of physical and emotional symptoms or problems and the specific essences that can be used to treat them.

To use this section, first find the presenting symptom and note the essence, or essences, recommended for it. You can then refer to Chapter 15 for a fuller description of the essences listed and identify those that seem most appropriate for the symptoms you want to treat. You do not necessarily need to use all the essences listed.

Please note that the essences suggested for each symptom are listed in alphabetical order, not in order of effectiveness.

The information contained in this repertory should be used only as a guide to the treatment of the symptoms listed. It cannot be claimed that the essences recommended will cure the condition in all cases. It is important that you consult a doctor or other health professional if symptoms persist.

Accidents

- Emergency Essence for pain, shock, stress and trauma, for everyday falls and bumps and also more serious injuries.

See also: Broken bones; Burns; Cuts

Addictions

- Boronia for the obsession related to addiction.
- Bottlebrush to help break the habit.
- Monga Waratah for a sense of your own strength.

Allergies

- Boab to dissolve family patterns.
- Bottlebrush and Boronia to reduce cravings.
- Bush Iris to drain away toxins from the body.
- Dagger Hakea to ease irritation and resentment.
- Fringed Violet to decrease sensitivity.
- Fringed Violet, Dagger Hakea and Bush Iris for hay fever.

See also: Food intolerance

Anger

- Dagger Hakea for resentment and bitterness towards family and friends.
- Mountain Devil for hatred, jealousy, suspicion.

Antibiotics

- Green Essence to reharmonise the digestive system.
- Purifying Essence to release any toxins after antibiotics.

Anxiety

- Dog Rose, the specific remedy for anxiety.
- Fringed Violet to clear any traumas.
- Hibbertia for hypervigilance.

Asthma

- Bush Iris for the lymphatic system and clearing excessive mucus and toxins from the sinuses, throat and lungs.
- Emergency Essence to release muscle spasms, ease terror and panic, and decrease sensitivity to environmental triggers.
- Purifying Essence to detoxify the body and to help remove any effects of cortisone creams or steroids.
- Tall Mulla Mulla specifically for the breath.

See also: Allergies; Bronchitis; Food intolerance; Rashes

Attention deficit hyperactivity disorder (ADHD)

- Black-eyed Susan to settle your child down and for impatience.
- Calm and Clear Essence for helping sleep and when they are too excited or scattered.
- Cognis Essence is very specific and excellent for treating this condition, for clarity and focus, and for integrating both sides of the brain.
- Kangaroo Paw to help your child be aware of others around them.

Autism

- Bauhinia for being open to the possibility of change.
- Boronia for obsession.
- Bush Fuchsia for a sense of orientation, to help speech.
- Dog Rose for fearfulness.
- Flannel Flower to help your child to trust and express their feelings.

- Freshwater Mangrove to help your child be open to new experiences.
- Kangaroo Paw to improve social skills and when too self-focused.
- Mountain Devil for hostility or aggression.
- Pink Flannel Flower to open up the heart chakra and help your child express and receive affection.
- Sundew to help your child feel grounded when confused.
- Wild Potato Bush for any frustration, which often triggers aggressive behaviour.
- Yellow Cowslip Orchid for a child who has to have and do things in a set order.

Bedwetting

- Billy Goat Plum for shame.
- Boab to release family patterns if the parents had the problem.
- Dog Rose for fear.
- Five Corners for confidence.
- Red Helmet Orchid for unresolved father issues or difficulties with authority figures.

Bites and stings

- Emergency Essence for pain and swelling, for allergic reactions and in the case of a more serious bite or sting, to calm your child until help arrives.

Biting or hitting other children

- Mountain Devil for any aggressive behaviour.
- Rough Bluebell if your child has a lack of empathy for others.
- Wild Potato Bush if your child is biting or hitting out of frustration.

Broken bones

- Emergency Essence for the pain, shock and trauma.
- Gymea Lily to heal ligaments and bones.
- Hibbertia to stimulate calcium production and speed up healing of the bone.

Bronchitis

- Bush Iris for mucus and congestion.
- Emergency Essence if your child is anxious or fearful because of the illness.
- Mulla Mulla for fever.
- Red Suva Frangipani for inflamed family situations.
- Sturt Desert Pea for grief and sadness.
- Tall Yellow Top for abandonment.

Bruises

- Emergency Essence for the initial trauma and pain.
- Tall Mulla Mulla for helping the integrity of the blood vessels.

Burns

- Solaris Essence, containing Mulla Mulla, to ease pain and minimise skin damage.

Cancer

- Bush Iris for fear of dying.
- Emergency Essence for pain relief.
- Kapok Bush if your child feels it's too hard and wants to give up.

- Mulla Mulla if your child is having radiation therapy, to minimise side effects.
- Purifying Essence to purify the organs of elimination, to purify emotions and to release toxicity in the case of chemotherapy.
- Southern Cross for feelings of 'Why me?' and 'It's not fair'.
- Transition Essence to ease fear and bring calm and serenity if a child is dying, making it easier to pass over.

Chicken pox

- Billy Goat Plum for feeling disgusted about scabs or rash.
- Emergency Essence for frustration and the discomfort of itchy skin.
- Spinifex to ease itchy blisters.
- Wild Potato Bush for the frustration of feeling curtailed.

Clinginess

- Confid Essence for insecurity and lack of confidence.
- Emergency Essence for acute episodes.

Colds

- Bush Fuchsia rubbed on bone behind the ear for sore ears.
- Calm and Clear Essence if your child has been feeling run down and stressed just before the cold.
- Emergency Essence for a sore throat, tenderness in the ears and coughs.
- Solaris Essence for fever.

See also: Coughs; Earache; Influenza; Sore throat.

Colic

- Calm and Clear Essence to help digestion.
- Emergency Essence cream rubbed on the stomach to ease pain.

Confidence

- Confid Essence to build confidence, for being true to yourself and doing what you need to do and easing anxiety and shyness.

Constipation

- Bottlebrush to clear the large intestine.
- Emergency Essence to help relax your child.

Coughs

- Bush Iris if the cough is wet.
- Emergency Essence rubbed below the sternum notch.
- Illawarra Flame Tree for feelings of rejection and a lowered immune system.
- Sturt Desert Pea for sadness.

See also: Bronchitis

Cuts

- Emergency Essence for shock.
- Slender Rice Flower for deeper cuts requiring stitches.
- Spinifex to heal fine cuts.

See also: Scars

Demanding behaviour

- Black-eyed Susan for impatience.
- Boronia for obsessive, nagging behaviour.
- Dog Rose for insecurity.
- Gymea Lily if your child wants to be the centre of attention, speaking over others.
- Isopogon for stubbornness.
- Kangaroo Paw if your child is unaware of the impact her behaviour is having on others.

Diabetes

- Peach-flowered Tea-tree to help balance the pancreas.

N.B. You will need to work in conjunction with your doctor.

Disinterest in food

- Black-eyed Susan to calm your child down.
- Jacaranda to help focus on eating.
- Sundew to help bring your child into the physical.

See also: Allergies; Food intolerance

Divorce

See: Separation or divorce of parents

Earache

- Bush Fuchsia for chronic ear infections internally and topically.
- Emergency Essence for the relief of pain.
- Mulla Mulla if fever is present.

Easily upset

- Emergency Essence for very sensitive children who are physic sponges, too sensitive to pain, frustration and feelings of rejection or unkindness.
- Space Clearing Essence to clear negative energy and create a harmonious environment.
- *See also:* Allergies; Food intolerance

Eczema

See: Rashes

Emotional pain

- Dog Rose for anxiety and insecurity.
- Five Corners for low self-esteem.
- Illawarra Flame Tree for rejection.
- Mountain Devil for anger.
- Sturt Desert Pea for grief.

Episiotomy

- Slender Rice Flower to ease tenderness and for faster healing.
- Wisteria, in Sexuality Essence, for feeling comfortable and confident with physical intimacy afterwards.

Falls

- Boab and Bush Fuchsia for any headaches.
- Emergency Essence to relax muscles and ease pain.

Important: Take your child to a doctor or hospital if there is any vomiting, loss of consciousness or persistent headache.

Fear

- Dog Rose for general fear and anxiety.
- Dog Rose of the Wild Forces for fear of losing control.
- Flannel Flower for fear of physical or emotional intimacy.
- Grey Spider Flower for terror and nightmares.
- Illawarra Flame Tree for fear of responsibility.
- Jacaranda for fear of making the wrong choice.
- Wedding Bush for fear of commitment.

Fear of others

- Dog Rose for anxiety and shyness.
- Fringed Violet for protection from 'bad' energy.

Febrile convulsions

- Emergency Essence given in frequent doses if convulsions start to help airways stay open and relax your child.
- Mulla Mulla to help prevent convulsions as well as reduce severity and frequency. Give at the first sign of fevers if there is a history of convulsions.

Fevers

- Mulla Mulla to ease fever and a burning sensation.
- She Oak to hydrate your child.

Important: Take your child to a doctor or hospital if his eyes appear at all sunken, his fever gets to over 40°, or if his skin is greyish.

Food intolerance

- Bauhinia for good functioning of the ileocaecal valve.
- Black-eyed Susan to slow down while eating.

- Boab to clear family patterns.
- Bottlebrush for irritable bowel syndrome and diarrhoea.
- Calm and Clear Essence for headaches, colic and hyperactivity.
- Dagger Hakea to help the gall bladder and with the production of bile.
- Emergency Essence when the reaction first occurs for headaches and gut problems.
- Jacaranda if your child is scattered and unfocused.
- Peach-flowered Tea-tree for the proper absorption of nutrients and to settle mood swings.
- Purifying Essence for skin rashes.

Frustration

- Black-eyed Susan for impatience.
- Wild Potato Bush for feeling burdened by the physical body and your child not being able to do what they want.

Fussy eater

- Bauhinia to help your child be open to something a bit different or something she is not used to eating.
- Freshwater Mangrove if your child has made up her mind about a food without even trying it.
- Paw Paw and Crowea to stimulate the appetite and aid digestion.

See also: Disinterest in food; Food intolerance

Gastric reflux

- Jacaranda to help digestive juices stay down.

German measles

- Emergency Essence for pain or discomfort.
- Mulla Mulla for fever.
- Wild Potato Bush for frustration about physical restrictions.

Glue ear

See: Earache

Grief

- Emergency Essence for initial shock after the news of an unexpected death or a bad prognosis.
- Fringed Violet if your child is picking up on others' pain, suffering and sadness.
- Red Suva Frangipini for ending relationships, the initial sadness and emotional intensity at the loss of a loved one, or for a child moving away from friends.
- Sturt Desert Pea for unresolved grief and sadness.
- Transition Essence to help ease the fear of death and to help prepare for and later cope with loss.

Hay fever

See: Allergies

Headaches

- Bottlebrush if your child is constipated.
- Calm and Clear Essence cream rubbed into the temples for a stress headache (it clears it very quickly).

- Emergency Essence if a headache follows a fall.
- Tall Yellow Top for chronic neck pain.

Head injuries

- Emergency Essence for pain, discomfort and loss of consciousness.
- Spinifex for damaged nerve endings.

Important: Take your child to a doctor or hospital if there is a loss of consciousness or there are any signs of vomiting or a headache lasting more than four hours.

Head lice

- Billy Goat Plum for feeling dirty or unclean or for shame and embarrassment.
- Green Essence internally and topically to remove parasites.
- Kapok Bush for the feeling that it's too hard and wanting to give up.

Hyperactivity

See: Attention deficit hyperactivity disorder

Hypervigilance

- Calm and Clear Essence if your child is tense or uptight.
- Hibbertia if your child is always on guard and never relaxed.
- Little Flannel Flower for more playfulness and fun.
- Mountain Devil for suspicious children who are not trusting.
- Sexuality Essence if there has been sexual or physical abuse or for feelings of not being safe in the past.

Influenza

- Black-eyed Susan for getting sick from doing too much.
- Bush Iris for the lymphatics.
- Green Essence to stop excess yeast and mould due to antibiotic use.
- Illawarra Flame Tree to boost the immune system.
- Jacaranda for children who get sick when they are too scattered with their energy.
- Mulla Mulla for fevers.
- Paw Paw for children who get sick when overwhelmed.

Learning difficulties

- Bush Fuchsia to integrate both hemispheres of the brain, dyslexia and ADD.
- Cognis Essence for focus, integration of information and attention to detail.

See also: Attention deficit hyperactivity disorder

Loss of a parent

- Bottlebrush for the loss of a mother.
- Red Helmet Orchid for the loss of a father.
- Red Suva Frangipani for the initial shock and trauma.
- Sturt Desert Rose for guilt.

See also: Grief

Low blood sugar levels

- Peach-flowered Tea-tree to stabilise blood sugar levels.

Manipulative behaviour

- Rough Bluebell to let go of manipulative behaviour and the hurting of others.

Mastitis

- Bush Iris for the lymphatic system.
- Emergency Essence cream to ease pain in the breast area.
- Mulla Mulla for heat, burning sensations and fever.
- Woman Essence for hormonal balance.

Measles

- Bush Iris for the lymphatic glands and to ease a cough.
- Emergency Essence to ease pain or distress.
- Green Essence as a gargle for a sore throat.
- Mulla Mulla to ease fever.

Morning sickness

- Calm and Clear Essence to settle your stomach and aid digestion.
- Confid Essence to ease any fear.
- Dagger Hakea to help the liver and reduce nausea.
- Woman Essence for hormonal balance.

Mumps

- Emergency Essence to ease pain or distress.
- Flannel Flower to protect a boy's testes.
- Hibbertia to ease swelling of the the parotid glands.
- Mulla Mulla to ease fever.

Nail biting

- Boronia and Bottlebrush together to break the habit.
- Crowea to settle nerves and stop worrying.
- Dog Rose for being anxious and fearful.

Nappy rash

- Emergency Essence drops and cream to ease a rash.
- Green Essence to purify.
- Purifying Essence to release toxins causing the rash.
- Spinifex applied topically to ease the rash.

Nightmares

- Dog Rose of the Wild Forces for intense fear.
- Green Spider Orchid for nightmares from past-life experiences.
- Grey Spider Flower for terror.
- Space Clearing Essence to clear unpleasant energies.

Night terrors

- Emergency Essence for terror and the altered state.

Nosebleeds

- Fringed Violet for psychic protection.
- Illawarra Flame Tree for emotional triggers.

Out of sorts

- Crowea to re-establish balance when feeling not quite right and as a general tonic.
- Dynamis Essence for vitality.

Poor bonding

- Bottlebrush for the mother–child bond.
- Flannel Flower for ease with physical intimacy.
- Red Helmet Orchid for the father–child bond.
- Tall Yellow Top for a sense of separation or loneliness.

Premature baby

- Bottlebrush to help the mother–child bond.
- Tall Mulla Mulla to treat possible asthma or bronchial problems.

Rashes

- Confid Essence if your child's self-confidence is affected by a rash.
- Emergency Essence cream. Apply after Green Essence, applied topically, has dried.
- Green Essence applied topically as a misting spray. Leave to dry.
- Purifying Essence to eliminate built-up toxins from the body.
- Solaris Essence if there are any heat or burning sensations.

Scars

- Slender Rice Flower to clear scarring, release emotion stored in the scar and to allow the energy to fully flow along any meridian that the scar crosses.

Separation anxiety

- Bauhinia and Bottlebrush to help your child be open to change ahead.
- Bottlebrush to strengthen the mother–child bond.
- Dog Rose for feelings of insecurity and for courage and confidence.
- Emergency Essence for distress at separation.
- Illawarra Flame Tree for a sense of rejection.
- Monga Waratah for dependence and clinginess.

Separation or divorce of parents
(many of these remedies would help parents too)

- Bauhinia to accept change that is about to happen i.e. parents divorcing and new step-family situations.
- Bottlebrush for strengthening the relationship with the mother and for change and upheaval.
- Cognis Essence to help to stay focused at school and with children's studies.
- Confid Essence for self-esteem.
- Dagger Hakea for resentment or any intense or negative feelings.
- Fringed Violet to help protect from any emotions of the parents.
- Illawarra Flame Tree for feelings of rejection.
- Little Flannel Flower to keep your child playful and fun loving and to prevent her assuming the burden of taking on the role of the other parent and growing up too quickly.
- Monga Waratah for having lost one parent and becoming clingy towards the other.
- Mountain Devil for anger.
- Red Helmet Orchid for strengthening the relationship with the father.
- Red Suva Frangipani for strength to cope and for rawness and turmoil.
- Rough Bluebell to prevent your child playing one parent off against the other.

- Southern Cross for sense of unfairness or for feeling life is unfair.
- Sturt Desert Rose for feelings of guilt.

See also: Grief

Sharing

- Bluebell for generosity and joyful sharing and resolving the belief that there is not enough.
- Bush Iris for an over-attachment to material things if your child is over five years of age and still not willing to share.
- Kangaroo Paw for a greater awareness of others and their needs.

Shyness

- Dog Rose to build courage and confidence.
- Five Corners to raise self-esteem and self-love.

Sibling rivalry

- Black-eyed Susan for impatience with a sibling.
- Dagger Hakea when resentment is building up that can explode.
- Five Corners for a child who always tries to be 'the good one' and always tries to please his parents and to boost self-esteem or for feeling bad about himself because he can't do what the sibling can, and for feeling not as important.
- Illawarra Flame Tree for feelings of rejection, wanting a lot of physical contact and bursting into tears.
- Mountain Devil where there is jealously of another sibling, aggression and lashing out physically.
- Pink Flannel Flower to help your child see the positive.
- Rough Bluebell for deliberately getting siblings into trouble or extreme cruelty/violence.

- Southern Cross when a child feels badly done by or feels that a sibling is getting more.
- Wild Potato Bush for extreme frustration at not being able to do what the older sibling is able to do.
- Yellow Cowslip Orchid if your child is judgmental or overly critical of a sibling.

Skinned knees

- Emergency Essence to speed up healing and for pain and shock.

Sleeping problems

- Bottlebrush for transition out of day naps.
- Bush Fuchsia to restore natural rhythms.
- Bush Iris to regulate body clock.
- Calm and Clear Essence to settle your child.
- Space Clearing Essence to clear energies in a bedroom.

Sore throat

- Bush Fuchsia to help verbal expression.
- Bush Iris to help the lymphatic system.
- Dynamis Essence if your child gets a sore throat from being run down and tired.
- Flannel Flower to help say and express one's feelings—not doing so can lead to this illness.
- Mulla Mulla for fever.

Spaced out

- Emergency Essence to relieve any earlier trauma especially head injuries.
- Purifying Essence if drugs were used during pregnancy or birth.
- Sexuality Essence if there has been sexual abuse.
- Sundew to ground a child who is vague and dreamy and for increased attention to detail and paying attention.

Sunburn

- Mulla Mulla to reduce the effects of the sun.
- Solaris Essence sprayed on sunburn to ease pain and stop peeling.

Surgery

- Emergency Essence before and after to help healing, for pain and discomfort and for fear and anxiety.
- Macrocarpa for the adrenal glands after anaesthetic.
- Purifying Essence to clear toxins after anaesthetic.
- Slender Rice Flower for healing any scars and healing meridians cut by incision.

Tantrums

- Calm and Clear Essence for impatience that leads to tantrums and for a sense of being overwhelmed by different emotions.
- Emergency Essence to settle your child, for a sense of losing control and for fear and confusion.
- Isopogon for stubbornness.
- Mountain Devil for rage.
- Red Helmet Orchid if your child is rebellious against authority and authority figures.

- Rough Bluebell for manipulation.
- Wild Potato Bush for frustration.

Teething

- Emergency Essence to ease pain, clear panic and fear, give staying power and for peace and calm.
- Solaris Essence for fever associated with teething.

Threat of miscarriage

- Emergency Essence to help prevent anything acute occurring.
- Woman Essence for the first trimester.

Travel sickness

- Crowea, Emergency Essence and Paw Paw—all three will help with nausea and other symptoms of motion sickness.
- Travel Essence taken hourly on plane trips to dramatically reduce jet lag and other stressful effects of flying. This remedy can be taken immediately before travel and every twenty minutes for motion sickness.

Vomiting

- Bottlebrush to help let go as vomiting is often the body trying to eliminate waste or get rid of things it doesn't want.
- Crowea and Paw Paw for any associated nausea.
See also: Morning sickness

Walking on tiptoe

- Cognis Essence for coordination and to ground your child.

Warts

- Five Corners and Billy Goat Plum for any dislike of the self, which is often the trigger for warts.
- Green Essence to shrink the warts.

Whingeing

- Dog Rose for fear and anxiety.
- Rough Bluebell for manipulation.
- Southern Cross for a sense of being a victim.

Worms

- Green Essence to clear parasites.
- Purifying Essence, which contains Bottlebrush, to detoxify the large intestine.

X-rays

- Mulla Mulla, found in Solaris Essence and Electro Essence, to reduce the absorption of radiation.

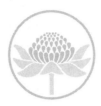

15

INDIVIDUAL ESSENCES

This section lists the negative (–) and positive (+) aspects of each essence. The negatives are conditions that the specific essences can treat, while the positives are the outcomes that the essence can bring about, enchance or help achieve. For example, Five Corners can be used to treat low self-esteem while also enhancing feelings of self-acceptance.

1. Alpine Mint Bush

— Mental and emotional exhaustion; lack of joy and weight of responsibility of care givers.

+ Revitalisation; joy; renewal.

2. Angelsword

— Interference with true spiritual connection to higher self; spiritual possession; spiritual confusion.

+ Spiritual discernment; ability to access gifts from past lifetimes; release of negatively held psychic energies; clear spiritual communication; psychic protection.

3. Banksia Robur

- − Disheartenment; lethargy; frustration; tiredness.
- + Enjoyment of life; enthusiasm; interest in life.

4. Bauhinia

- − Resistance to change; rigidity; reluctance.
- + Acceptance; open-mindedness.

5. Billy Goat Plum

- − Shame; inability to accept the physical self; physical loathing.
- + Sexual pleasure and enjoyment; acceptance of self and one's physical body; open-mindedness.

6. Black-eyed Susan

- − Impatience; being 'on the go' or over-committed; constant striving.
- + Ability to turn inward and be still; slowing down; inner peace.

7. Bluebell

- − Being closed; fear of lack; greed; rigidity.
- + Opening the heart; belief in abundance; universal trust; joyful sharing; unconditional love.

8. Boab

- − Enmeshment in negative family patterns; for recipients of abuse and prejudice.
- + Personal freedom by releasing family patterns; clearing of other, non-family, negative karmic connections.

9. Boronia

- — Obsessive thoughts; pining; suffering a broken heart.
- + Clarity; serenity; creative visualisation.

10. Bottlebrush

- — Unresolved mother issues; feeling overwhelmed by major life changes: old age, adolescence, parenthood, pregnancy, approaching death.
- + Serenity and calmness; ability to cope and move on; mother–child bonding; balancing large intestine.

11. Bush Fuchsia

- — Being switched off; nervousness about public speaking; ignoring gut feelings; clumsiness.
- + Having the courage to speak out; clarity; being in touch with intuition; integration of information; integration of male and female aspects; coordination; balancing ear and voice.

12. Bush Gardenia

- — Stale relationships; self-interest; unawareness.
- + Passion; renewal of interest in partner; improvement in communication.

13. Bush Iris

- — Fear of death; materialism; atheism; physical excess; avarice.
- + Awakening of spirituality; acceptance of death as a transitional state; clearance of blocks in the base chakra and trust centre; balancing the lymphatic system.

14. Christmas Bell

- — Lack of abundance; sense of lack; poor stewardship of one's possessions.
- + Help in manifesting desired outcomes; assistance with mastery of the physical plane.

15. Crowea

- — Continual worrying; a sense of being 'not quite right'.
- + Peace and calmness; balance and centring of the individual; clarity of one's feelings; balancing the stomach, muscles and tendons.

16. Dagger Hakea

- — Resentment; bitterness towards close family, friends and lovers.
- + Forgiveness; open expression of feelings; balancing the liver and gall bladder.

17. Dog Rose

- — Fearfulness; shyness; insecurity; apprehension with other people; niggling fears.
- + Confidence; belief in self; courage; ability to embrace life more fully; balancing the kidneys.

18. Dog Rose of the Wild Forces

- — Fear of losing control; hysteria; pain with no apparent cause.
- + Feeling calm and centred in times of inner and outer turmoil; emotional balance.

19. Five Corners

- − Low self-esteem; dislike of self; a crushed, held-in personality; drab and colourless clothing.
- + Love and acceptance of self; celebration of own beauty; joyousness.

20. Flannel Flower

- − Dislike of being touched; lack of sensitivity in males; being uncomfortable with intimacy.
- + Gentleness and sensitivity in touching; trust; openness; expression of feelings; joy in physical activity.

21. Freshwater Mangrove

- − Heart closure due to expectations or prejudices that have been taught, not personally experienced.
- + Openness to new experiences, people and perceptual shifts; healthy questioning of traditional standards and beliefs.

22. Fringed Violet

- − Damage to aura; distress; lack of psychic protection.
- + Removal of effects of recent or old distressing events; healing of damage to aura; psychic protection.

23. Green Spider Orchid

- − Nightmares and phobias from past-life experiences; intense negative reactions to the sight of blood.
- + Telepathic communication; ability to withhold information until timing is appropriate; attunement.

24. Grey Spider Flower

- — Terror; fear of supernatural and psychic attack; nightmares.
- + Faith; calmness; courage.

25. Gymea Lily

- — Arrogance; attention seeking; craving of status and glamour; a dominating and over-riding personality.
- + Humility; allowing others to express themselves and contribute; awareness, appreciation and taking notice of others; specific action on the spine, bones and ligaments.

26. Hibbertia

- — Fanaticism about self-improvement; drive to acquire knowledge; excessive self-discipline; superiority; hypervigilance.
- + Contentment with own knowledge; acceptance; ownership and utilisation of own knowledge.

27. Illawarra Flame Tree

- — Overwhelming sense of rejection; fear of responsibility.
- + Confidence; commitment; self-reliance; self-approval.

28. Isopogon

- — Inability to learn from past experience; stubbornness; a controlling personality.
- + Ability to learn from past experience; retrieval of forgotten skills; being able to relate without manipulating or controlling; ability to remember the past.

29. Jacaranda

- — Feeling scattered, changeable, dithering, in a rush.
- + Decisiveness; quick thinking; centredness.

30. Kangaroo Paw

- — Gaucheness; unawareness; insensitivity; ineptiness; clumsiness.
- + Kindness; sensitivity; savoir-faire; enjoyment of people; relaxation.

31. Kapok Bush

- — Apathy; resignation; discouragement; half-heartedness.
- + Willingness; application; wanting to 'give it a go'; persistence; perception.

32. Little Flannel Flower

- — Denial of the 'child' within; seriousness in children; grimness in adults.
- + Carefreeness; playfulness; joy.

33. Macrocarpa

- — Feeling drained, jaded, worn out.
- + Enthusiasm; inner strength; endurance.

34. Mint Bush

- — Perturbation; confusion; spiritual emergence; initial turmoil and feeling void of spiritual initiation.
- + Smooth spiritual initiation; clarity; calmness; ability to cope.

35. Monga Waratah

— Neediness; co-dependency; inability to do things alone; disempowerment; an addictive personality.

+ Strengthening of one's will; reclaiming of one's spirit; belief that one can break the dependency of any behaviour, substance or person; self-empowerment.

36. Mountain Devil

— Hatred; anger; holding grudges; suspiciousness.

+ Unconditional love; happiness; healthy boundaries; forgiveness.

37. Mulla Mulla

— Fear of flames and hot objects; distress associated with exposure to heat and sun; burns; fever.

+ Reduction in the effects of fire and sun; feeling comfortable with fire and heat.

38. Old Man Banksia

— Weariness; phlegmatic personalities; disheartenment; frustration.

+ Enjoyment of life; renewal of enthusiasm; interest in life.

39. Paw Paw

— Sense of being overwhelmed; inability to resolve problems; feeling burdened by decision.

+ Improved access to higher self for problem solving; assimilation of new ideas; calmness; clarity.

40. Peach-flowered Tea-tree

- — Mood swings; lack of commitment to follow through projects; being easily bored; hypochondria; sugar cravings and imbalances.
- + Ability to complete projects; personal stability; taking responsibility for one's health.

41. Philotheca

- — Inability to accept acknowledgment; excessive generosity.
- + Ability to receive love and acknowledgment; ability to let in praise.

42. Pink Flannel Flower

- — Feeling of life being dull and flat; lack of joy or appreciation for the everyday aspects of life.
- + Gratitude; joie de vivre; keeping open one's heart chakra; appreciation.

43. Pink Mulla Mulla

- — Deep ancient wounds on the psyche; assuming an outer guarded and prickly persona to prevent being hurt; keeping people at a distance.
- + Deep spiritual healing; trusting and opening up.

44. Red Grevillea

- — Feeling stuck; oversensitiveness; being affected by criticism and unpleasant people; too much reliance on others.
- + Boldness; strength to leave unpleasant situations; indifference to the judgement of others.

45. Red Helmet Orchid

- − Rebelliousness; hot-headedness; unresolved father issues; selfishness.
- + Father–child bonding; sensitivity; respect; consideration.

46. Red Lily

- − Vagueness; disconnectedness; feeling split; lack of focus; daydreaming.
- + Feeling grounded; focus; living in the present; connection with life and God.

47. Red Suva Frangipani

- − Initial grief, sadness and upset of either a relationship at rock bottom or of the death of a loved one; emotional upheaval, turmoil and rawness.
- + Feeling calm and nurtured; inner peace and strength to cope.

48. Rough Bluebell

- − Being deliberately hurtful, manipulative, exploitive or malicious.
- + Compassion; release of one's inherent love vibration; sensitivity.

49. She Oak

- − Female imbalance; inability to conceive for non-physical reasons.
- + Emotional openness to conceive; female balance; hydration.

50. Silver Princess

- − Aimlessness; despondence; feeling flat; lacking direction.
- + Motivation; direction; life purpose.

51. Slender Rice Flower

- — Prejudice; racism; narrow-mindedness; comparison with others.
- + Humility; group harmony; cooperation; perception of beauty in others; healing of scars.

52. Southern Cross

- — Victim mentality; complaining; bitterness; martyrdom; poverty consciousness.
- + Personal power; taking responsibility; positiveness.

53. Spinifex

- — Sense of being a victim to illness; damage to nerves; fine cuts; blistering lesions.
- + Empowerment through emotional understanding of illness.

54. Sturt Desert Pea

- — Emotional pain; deep hurt; sadness.
- + Letting go; trigger for healthy grieving; release of deeply held grief and sadness.

55. Sturt Desert Rose

- — Guilt; regret and remorse; low self-esteem; being easily led.
- + Courage; conviction; being true to self; integrity.

56. Sundew

- — Vagueness; disconnectedness; feeling split; indecision; lack of focus; daydreaming.
- + Attention to detail; feeling grounded; focus; living in the present.

57. Sunshine Wattle

- — Feeling stuck in the past; expectation of a grim future; struggle.
- + Optimism; acceptance of the beauty and joy in the present; openness to a bright future.

58. Sydney Rose

- — Feeling separated, deserted, unloved or morbid.
- + Realising we are all one; feeling safe and at peace; heartfelt compassion; sense of unity.

59. Tall Mulla Mulla

- — Feeling ill at ease; fearfulness of circulating and mixing with others; being a loner; distress and avoidance of confrontation.
- + Feeling relaxed and secure with other people; encouragement of social interaction; balance of circulation.

60. Tall Yellow Top

- — Alienation; loneliness; isolation.
- + Sense of belonging; acceptance of self and others; knowing that you are 'home'; ability to reach out.

61. Turkey Bush

- — Experiencing a creative block; disbelief in own creative ability.
- + Inspired creativity; creative expression; focus; renewal of artistic confidence.

62. Waratah

- — Despair; hopelessness; inability to respond to a crisis.
- + Courage; tenacity; adaptability; strong faith; enhancement of survival skills.

63. Wedding Bush

- — Difficulty with commitment.
- + Commitment to relationships; commitment to goals; dedication to life purpose.

64. Wild Potato Bush

- — Feeling weighed down; feeling encumbered; heavy metal toxicity.
- + Ability to move on in life; freedom; renewal of enthusiasm.

65. Wisteria

- — Feeling uncomfortable with sex; being closed sexually; male machismo.
- + Sexual enjoyment; enhanced sensuality; sexual openness; gentleness.

66. Yellow Cowslip Orchid

- — Being critical, judgemental, bureaucratic, nit picking.
- + Expressing humanitarian concern; impartiality; being able to step back from emotions; constructiveness; a keener sense of arbitration.

COMPANION ESSENCES

67. Autumn Leaves

- — Difficulties in the transition of passing over from the physical plane to the spiritual world.
- + Letting go and moving on; increase of awareness and communication with loved ones in the spiritual world.

68. Green Essence

- — Emotional distress associated with intestinal and skin disorders.
- + Harmonising the vibration of any yeast, mould or parasite to one's own vibration; purification.

69. Lichen

- — Not knowing to look for and move into the Light when passing over; being Earth-bound in the astral plane.
- + Easement of one's transition into the Light; assistance in separation between the physical and the etheric bodies; release of Earth-bound energies.

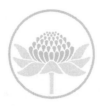

16

COMBINATON ESSENCES

All essences are available as drops only unless stated otherwise.

Abund Essence

- − Pessimism; being closed to receiving; fear of lack; poverty consciousness.
- + Joyful sharing; belief in abundance; clearing of financial sabotage patterns; universal trust.

Aids in releasing negative beliefs, family patterns, sabotage and fear of lack. In so doing, it allows you to be open to fully receiving great riches on all levels, not just financial.

Contains: Bluebell, Boab, Christmas Bell, Five Corners, Philotheca, Pink Flannel Flower, Southern Cross, Sunshine Wattle.

Adol Essence

- − Feeling of hopelessness; insensitivity; sense of not belonging; having an 'it's not fair' attitude; embarrassment; rebelliousness; anger.
- + Coping with change; consideration of others; enhancement of communication; improved self-esteem.

Addresses the major issues teenagers commonly experience. It enhances acceptance of self, communication, social skills, harmony in relationships, maturity, emotional stability and optimism.

Contains: Billy Goat Plum, Boab, Bottlebrush, Dagger Hakea, Five Corners, Flannel Flower, Kangaroo Paw, Red Helmet Orchid, Southern Cross, Sunshine Wattle, Tall Yellow Top.

Calm and Clear Essence
(also available as mist and cream)

- — Always feeling overcommitted; having no time for self; impatience; rushing; worry; poor sleeping patterns.
- + Encouraging own time and space; helping to wind down, relax and have fun; clarity, calmness and peace.

Helps to find time for one's self, to relax without external pressures and demands, to wind down and enjoy relaxing pursuits.

Contains: Black-eyed Susan, Bottlebrush, Boronia, Bush Fuchsia, Crowea, Jacaranda, Little Flannel Flower, Paw Paw.

Cognis Essence

- — Daydreaming; confusion; feeling overwhelmed.
- + Assimilation of ideas; clarity and focus; enhancement of all learning abilities and skills.

Gives clarity and focus when working, speaking, reading or studying. It balances the intuitive and cognitive processes and helps integrate ideas and information. Excellent for study or pursuits that require intense focus. It assists problem solving by improving access to the higher self, which stores all past knowledge and experiences.

Contains: Bush Fuchsia, Isopogon, Jacaranda, Paw Paw, Sundew.

Confid Essence

- − Low self-esteem; guilt; shyness; lack of conviction; victim mentality.
- + Taking of responsibility for one's life; integrity; confidence; personal power; being true to one's self.

Brings out the positive qualities of self-esteem and confidence. It allows us to feel comfortable around other people and resolve negative beliefs we may hold about ourselves as well as any guilt we may harbour from past actions. This combination also helps us take responsibility for situations and events that occur in our lives and to realise we have the ability and power not only to change those events, but also to create those we want.

Contains: Boab, Dog Rose, Five Corners, Southern Cross, Sturt Desert Rose.

Creative Essence

- − Creative blocks and inhibitions; difficulty expressing feelings.
- + Enhancement of singing; creative expression; clarity of voice; public speaking.

Inspires creative and emotional expression and gives courage and clarity in public speaking and singing. This essence frees the voice. It also helps to clear creative blocks and to find creative solutions in all of life's pursuits.

Contains: Bush Fuchsia, Crowea, Five Corners, Flannel Flower, Red Grevillea, Tall Mulla Mulla, Turkey Bush.

Dynamis Essence

- − Temporary loss of drive, enthusiasm and excitement.
- + Renewal of passion and enthusiasm for life; centring and harmonising of one's vital forces.

Renews enthusiasm and joy for life. It is for those who feel 'not quite right', drained, jaded or not fully recovered from setbacks.

Contains: Banksia Robur, Crowea, Illawarra Flame Tree, Macrocarpa, Old Man Banksia, Yellow Cowslip Orchid.

Electro Essence

- — Feeling drained and flat; feeling out of balance with Earth's rhythms.
- + Reduction of emotional and physical effects of all radiation.

Greatly relieves fear and distress associated with Earth, electrical and electromagnetic radiation. It helps to bring one into balance with the natural rhythms of the Earth.

Contains: Bush Fuchsia, Crowea, Fringed Violet, Mulla Mulla, Paw Paw, Waratah.

Emergency Essence
(also available as cream, mist and oral spray)

- — Panic; distress; fear; emotional or physical pain and upset.
- + Ability to cope.

Excellent for any emotional upset. It has a calming effect during a crisis. If a person needs specialised medical help, this essence will provide comfort until treatment is available. Administer this remedy every hour or more frequently if necessary, until the person feels better.

Contains: Angelsword, Crowea, Dog Rose of the Wild Forces, Fringed Violet, Grey Spider Flower, Sundew, Waratah. Creams only also include: Slender Rice Flower, Spinifex.

Face, Hand and Body Essence
(cream only)

— Dislike of physical self, body, skin texture and touch.

+ Acceptance of physical body; love and nurturing of self; hydration of the skin.

Encourages love, nurturing, care and touch of your physical body. Helps to deal with any dislike and non-acceptance of one's body, skin texture or intimate loving touch.

Contains: Billy Goat Plum, Five Corners, Flannel Flower, Little Flannel Flower, Mulla Mulla, She Oak, Wisteria.

Meditation Essence

— Poor quality meditation; psychic attack; damaged aura; feeling psychically drained.

+ Awakening of spirituality; enhancement of intuition; inner guidance; help in accessing higher self; deeper meditation; telepathy.

Awakens one's spirituality and allows one to go deeper into any religious or spiritual practice. Enhances access to the higher self while providing psychic protection and healing of the aura. Highly recommended for anyone practising meditation.

Contains: Angelsword, Boronia, Bush Fuchsia, Bush Iris, Fringed Violet, Green Spider Orchid, Red Lily.

Purifying Essence

— Emotional and physical toxicity; feeling encumbered; emotional baggage.

+ Sense of release and relief; feeling spring cleaned.

Releases and clears emotional waste and residual by-products, and clears built-up emotional baggage.

Contains: Bauhinia, Bottlebrush, Bush Iris, Dagger Hakea, Dog Rose, Wild Potato Bush.

Relationship Essence

- − Emotional pain and turmoil; confusion; resentment; feeling blocked, held-in emotions; inabilty to relate.
- + Expressing feelings; enhanced communication; forgiveness; breaking of negative family conditioning; renewal of interest; enhancement of parent−child bonding.

Enhances the quality of all relationships, especially intimate ones. It clears and releases resentment, blocked emotions and the confusion, emotional pain and turmoil of a rocky relationship. Helps one verbalise and express feelings and improve communication. This essence breaks any early negative family conditioning and patterns that affect us in our current adult relationships. For those in intimate relationships, a perfect remedy to follow this combination is Sexuality Essence.

Contains: Bluebell, Boab, Bottlebrush, Bush Gardenia, Dagger Hakea, Flannel Flower, Mint Bush, Red Helmet Orchid, Red Suva Frangipani, Wedding Bush.

Sensuality Essence
(mist only)

- − Fear of emotional and physical intimacy.
- + Encouraging intimacy, passion and sensual fulfilment.

Encourages the ability to enjoy physical and emotional intimacy, passion and sensual fulfilment.

Contains: Bush Gardenia, Billy Goat Plum, Flannel Flower, Little Flannel Flower, Macrocarpa, Wisteria.

Sexuality Essence

- − Effects of sexual abuse; shame; feeling uptight about sexuality; fear of intimacy.
- + Renewal of passion; sensuality; enjoyment of touch and intimacy; playfulness; fulfilment.

Helpful for releasing shame and the effects of physical or sexual abuse and trauma. It allows one to feel comfortable with and to fully accept one's body. It enables the individual to be open to sensuality and touch and to enjoy physical and emotional intimacy. Sexuality Essence renews passion and interest in relationships.

Contains: Billy Goat Plum, Bush Gardenia, Flannel Flower, Fringed Violet, Little Flannel Flower, Sturt Desert Rose, Wisteria.

Solaris Essence

- − Fear and distress associated with fire.
- + Reduction of the negative effects of fire and the sun's rays.

Greatly relieves fear and distress associated with fire, heat and sun. An excellent remedy to have handy during summer and long exposure to the sun.

Contains: Mulla Mulla, She Oak, Spinifex.

Space Clearing Essence
(mist only)

- − Negative mental, emotional and psychic energies; disharmonious or unpleasant environments.
- + Enhancement of sacred space; clearing of negative and psychic energies; creation of safe, harmonious environments; allowing one to feel still and reflective.

Creates sacred, safe and harmonious environments. Purifies and releases environments of built-up negative emotional, mental and psychic energies. Great for clearing tense situations and environments and restoring balance.

Contains: Angelsword, Boab, Fringed Violet, Lichen, Red Lily.

Transition Essence

- — Feeling stuck; lack of direction; fear of death; fear of the unknown; non-acceptance.
- + Acceptance of change; serenity; easing fear of death; passing over in peace.

Helps one to cope and move through any major life change. It brings about an awareness of one's life direction, especially for people who are at a crossroad. Alternatively, those who know what they want but do not know how to achieve it will benefit from this combination. It also eases the fear of death as well as helping one come to terms with it. This remedy, consequently, allows one to easily and gently pass over with calmness, dignity and serenity.

Contains: Autumn Leaves, Bauhinia, Bottlebrush, Bush Iris, Lichen, Mint Bush, Red Grevillea, Silver Princess.

Travel Essence
(also available as mist and cream)

- — Disorientation; feeling personally depleted and drained; emotional effects of travel; jet lag; motion sickness.
- + Refreshment; centring; maintenance of sense of personal space.

Addresses the problems encountered with jet travel. It enables a person to arrive at their destination feeling balanced and ready to go. The use of this essence is beneficial for all forms of travel.

Contains: Banksia Robur, Bottlebrush, Bush Fuchsia, Bush Iris, Crowea, Fringed Violet, Macrocarpa, Mulla Mulla, Paw Paw, Red Lily, She Oak, Silver Princess, Sundew, Tall Mulla Mulla.

Woman Essence
(also available as mist and cream)

- − Mood swings; weariness; physical dislike; female hormonal imbalances.
- + Female balance; calmness and stability; helping to cope with change.

Harmonises any imbalances during menstruation and menopause. It allows a woman to discover and feel good about herself, her own body and her beauty.

Contains: Billy Goat Plum, Bottlebrush, Bush Fuchsia, Crowea, Five Corners, Mulla Mulla, Old Man Banksia, Peach-flowered Tea-tree, Pink Flannel Flower, She Oak.

Bibliography

Allen, Hannah, *Don't Get Stuck*, Natural Hygiene Press, Florida, 1985

Biddulph, Steve, *Raising Boys*, Finch Publishing, Sydney, 1998

Dethlefsen, Thorwald & Dahlke, Rudiger, *The Healing Power Of Illness*, Element Books, Dorset, 1990

Green, Dr Christopher, *Toddler Taming*, Doubleday, Sydney, 1990

Gruner, Mark & Brown, Eric, *Your Numbers Your Life*, John Bannister Results, Maroochydore, 1995

Hay, Louise, *You Can Heal Your Life*, Hay House, Santa Monica, 1984

Losey, Meg Blackburn, *The Children of Now*, New Page Books, Franklin Lakes, NJ, 2007

Miller, Neil Z., *Vaccines, Autism and Childhood Disorders*, New Atlantean Press, Santa Fe, 2003

Noontil, Annette, *The Body is the Barometer of the Soul*, Noontil, Melbourne, 1994

Odent, Michel, *Birth Reborn*, Pantheon Books, New York, 1984

Parker, Jan & Stimpson, Jan, *Raising Happy Children*, Hodder & Staunton, London, 1999

Phillips, Dr David A., *Discovering the Inner Self*, Hay House, Sydney, 1996

Ray, Sondra, *Ideal Birth*, Celestial Arts, San Francisco, 1985

Ray, Sondra & Mandel, Bob, *Birth & Relationships*, Celestial Arts, California, 1987

Rossmanith, Angela, *When Will the Children Play?*, Reed Books, Melbourne, 1997

Stevenson, Ian, *Children Who Remember Past Lives: A question of reincarnation*, University Press, Virginia, 1987

Thomas, Jan, *Chiron . . . on Children*, Cheironia, Ballarat, 2001

Verny, T., *The Secret Life of the Unborn Child*, Sphere Books, London, 1981

Virtue, Doreen, *The Crystal Children*, Hay House, Sydney, 2003

White, Ian, *Australian Bush Flower Essences*, Bantam Books, Sydney, 1991

——*Bush Flower Healing*, Random House, Sydney, 1999

——*White Light Essences*, Australian Bush Flower Essences, Sydney, 2002

Contact details

AUSTRALIAN BUSH FLOWER ESSENCES

For further information on our ever-evolving and expanding range of products, including the White Light CD and our soon to be released Pregnancy, Labour, Children and Parent range of essences, please contact our office or website.

Australian Bush Flower Essences
45 Booralie Road
Terrey Hills NSW 2084
Australia

Telephone: (02) 9450 1388 International: 61+2 9450 1388
Facsimilie: (02) 9450 2866 International: 61+2 9450 2866
Email: info@ausflowers.com.au
Website: www.ausflowers.com.au

THE AUSTRALIAN BUSH FLOWER ESSENCE SOCIETY

The society has been formed to provide you with the most up-to-date information on Bush Essences. There is a minimal annual subscription fee, for which members receive four newsletters per year containing updates on essences, details of workshops and many special offers. It will also allow you a forum, through the publication of case histories, to share your knowledge and experience of flower essences.

We are always happy to receive any case histories or testimonials; your contributions are greatly valued.

Contact details for the society are as above.